Arts Therapies in Psychiatric Rehabilitation

Umberto Volpe
Editor

Arts Therapies in Psychiatric Rehabilitation

Springer

Editor
Umberto Volpe
Chair of Psychiatry
Department of Neurosciences/DIMSC
Università Politecnica delle Marche
Ancona
Italy

ISBN 978-3-030-76207-0 ISBN 978-3-030-76208-7 (eBook)
https://doi.org/10.1007/978-3-030-76208-7

This Springer imprint is published by the registered company Springer Nature Switzerland AG
The registered company address is: Gewerbestrasse 11, 6330 Cham, Switzerland

Foreword

Arts and arts therapies have played a major role in the history and development of modern psychiatry.

When large asylums were established in the nineteenth century, they were originally designed to provide a dignified and therapeutic environment. Within decades however most of them became overcrowded and conditions significantly deteriorated. In this situation, at various places patients in these asylums were permitted or at times even encouraged to engage in arts activities, mainly drawing and painting. Intended as an occupation to interrupt the everyday boredom, in some places it amounted to more. At the end of the nineteenth century, Emil Kraepelin at the University of Heidelberg had started a collection of art produced by patients. In 1919, Hans Prinzhorn, a psychiatrist who had also graduated in art history, was employed to expand the collection including pieces created in other asylums. The collection, which today is housed in its own museum in Heidelberg, soon had 5000 works created by about 450 patients. When published in a book with illustrations [1], the collection was appreciated for its unusual artistic value by arts critics and led to surprise, curiosity and respect for the mentally ill in the public. This demonstration of the creativity of patients in asylums is likely to have contributed to calls for reforms of the asylums which became stronger from the 1920s onwards.

Whilst arts works done by psychiatric patients influenced how the public viewed and respected the patients, over time arts activities became even more important and were part of the reforms of the mainly custodial form of care that was provided in the asylums. Nise da Silveira graduated in medicine in Brazil in 1926, as one of the first female medical doctors in the country. She qualified in psychiatry and was strictly opposed to electroconvulsive therapy, lobotomy and insulin therapy as the prevailing forms of psychiatric treatments at the time. In the 1930s, she spent 18 months as a political prisoner. When she returned to psychiatry she established an occupational therapy unit at Brazil's largest psychiatric hospital in Rio de Janeiro where she encouraged patients to engage in arts activities, mainly painting and modelling [2]. In 1952, she founded the 'Museum of Images of the Unconscious' in which the arts works by patients were and still are exhibited. The arts activities promoted by Nise da Silveira were not formal therapies. Originally they had two aims, i.e. to provide meaningful occupation to patients and to open up new ways to explore and understand their experiences, particularly the unconscious of their minds [3]. The latter interest focused on patients with psychotic disorders and was influenced by and associated with Jungian psychoanalysis. However, arts activities soon became part of an emancipatory process for the patients. In 1956, Nise da Silveira established the 'Casa de Palmeiras' (House of the Palm Trees) where patients who had left the asylum attended voluntarily, spent time together and focused on free expressions of their art, which included paintings over the walls and doors of the building [4].

Hans Prinzhorn and Nise da Silveira were prominent protagonists in championing the role of arts in the history of psychiatry. Many other initiatives are less well known. Yet, the practice of engaging patients in arts activities became increasingly widespread when reform ideas gained momentum in mental health care after the Second World War. Different art forms were used, including a range of visual arts, but also various forms of music, dance and drama. All this happened very inconsistently, usually driven and sustained by the initiative of individuals, mostly clinicians but also artists without any clinical qualification. Over time, mental health care reforms were initiated in practically all high-income countries, although time of onset, political drivers, processes, pace and exact outcomes varied substantially across countries. Old-fashioned asylums were abolished or downsized. Smaller inpatient units attached to general hospitals and alternative services such as day hospitals and drop-in centres in the community were established. The treatment programmes in all these services—from the remaining asylums to the new acute inpatient departments and community-based services—commonly included some form of arts activities. Providing such activities on a mere outpatient basis in the community was less common initially. One possible reason is that these arts activities were typically organised in groups, and attending groups can be more difficult for outpatients who have to go somewhere specifically for that group activity than for patients who spend much time in the building where the group is provided anyway. Since the 1950s, as arts activities increasingly had an explicit therapeutic aspiration, more specified forms of formalised art therapies were developed using different underlying therapeutic models, and formal qualifications for arts therapists with defined curricula were established.

Today, there is a wide range of arts therapies which in practice are provided in very different ways, as individual and group therapies—the latter as open or closed groups—over varying periods of time, with sessions of different lengths and frequencies, with different approaches for integrating verbal and non-verbal components, and obviously using different arts modalities. They are also based on or refer to very different theories and vary in their exact therapeutic aims, as outlined in other chapters in this book. Even when therapies share the same name (e.g. 'music therapy') they do not necessarily have much in common other than the main arts modality that has been chosen. Thus, it is difficult to arrive at general conclusions about the role of arts therapies in psychiatry at present. Still, it may be possible to make some overarching comments.

As illustrated, arts activities by patients were often part of a humanistic approach, focusing on patients' creative resources and skills rather than on their deficits [5], putting patients' own ideas and products at the centre of the therapeutic process, and potentially allowing others to see or hear the creations of patients with respect and admiration. This link between arts therapies and a humanistic approach in psychiatry does still exist, but can also lead to two types of criticism. One criticism is that arts therapies might potentially be paternalistic. Clinicians often come from a different social background than many of their patients and are likely to have had a different socialisation with more exposure to formal education in artistic skills. When providing arts therapies, clinicians may impose their own values and cultural beliefs on others, and ignore that these arts forms may not really appeal to or are seen as an appropriate form of self-expression by the patients. Another potential criticism may be based on concerns about the benefits of arts therapies. Are they—despite reflecting a humanistic approach and provided with best intentions—possibly without any tangible therapeutic effect? At times of economic pressure on mental health services, such scepticism can easily lead to cuts in the funding for arts therapies, and recently this has already happened in various services, e.g. in the National Health Service in the United Kingdom, although again very inconsistently.

A debate about the justification of funding for arts therapies leads to the question whether arts therapies are evidence-based and to what extent their therapeutic effect has been demonstrated in randomised controlled trials. The evidence for different arts therapies is reviewed in other chapters in this book. Overall, the literature seems to suggest that there is some evidence for the effectiveness of different forms of arts therapies, but that most studies have methodological shortcomings and that more rigorous studies are required. A potential criticism even of positive findings is that most trials in arts therapies were led and conducted by arts therapists themselves, potentially leading to a conflict of interests, and that more studies should be run by independent researchers with no personal interest in a positive or negative result. Nevertheless, the existing evidence appears encouraging and not worse than for many other psycho-social treatments. At the same time, it needs to be considered that the three largest trials on different arts therapies—MATISSE [6], TIME-A [7] and NESS [8]—all failed to show a positive effect of arts therapies, albeit in very specific populations, i.e. children with autism and adult patients with schizophrenia. More high-quality trials will hopefully follow, but future research should be wider and consist not only of trials.

The dominating model of evidence-based medicine is to test a defined intervention for a defined diagnostic group. Studies on arts therapies should go beyond this, not just because the methodology of randomised controlled trials has well-documented limitations. There are further reasons: Firstly, one can hardly test all forms of arts therapies for every single diagnostic group in large and rigorous trials. There is not enough funding and research capacity for that, also considering that new forms of arts therapies may be developed in the future. Secondly, such trials require a clear definition and manualisation of the given intervention which comes with disadvantages: (a) the manualisation may hinder what is a major factor in these therapies, i.e. the improvisation and spontaneity in the encounter of human beings in the therapeutic context which cannot be manualised and may compromise any manual; (b) the strictly defined format required in a trial with a defined number of sessions of a defined length and frequency can make therapies stale and institutionally rigid. Thirdly and lastly, instead of regarding arts therapies as fixed methods to treat patients, they may be more appropriately seen as a context in which a specific form of art is used to engage patients and facilitate interactions and experiences that can help to reduce and overcome mental distress. Thus, processes and individual responses can vary, and a generalised statement as to whether a specific form of arts therapy is 'effective' or not would hardly reflect the real complexity of human relationships and experiences. As a consequence, more qualitative research on what actually happens in these therapies and how the arts are utilised in the process of overcoming mental distress is required to advance our understanding of how arts can be used to help psychiatric patients.

There are a number of reasons for a renewed and stronger interest in arts and arts therapies in psychiatry [9]. One of them is the failure of neuroscience and other psychiatric research to come up with new treatments that are clearly more effective than what was available 50 years ago. Thus, the challenge is to search for approaches that are different from pharmacotherapy and conventional talking therapies. In this context, arts therapies offer a potential for new developments and innovation, perhaps not for all patients, but possibly for many. For this, arts therapies may have to be less fixed in their format and use arts in a more flexible way to engage and help people with mental disorders than is envisaged in current formalised therapies. The label 'therapy' may not always be helpful in this. Arts have the potential to surprise, amuse, scare, enthuse, open up completely new perspectives, facilitate learning or rediscovering of skills, lead to unusual human encounters, and trigger all sorts of helpful therapeutic processes. The challenge is to utilise this huge potential so that people with mental distress benefit from it, in whatever form this may happen.

Arts and arts therapies had a positive influence in the history of psychiatry as much as their own development reflected wider changes in psychiatry. Given their potential to appeal and to widen human experience, they may have an even more central role in the future.

London, UK Stefan Priebe

References

1. Prinzhorn H. *Bildnerei der Geisteskranken. Ein Beitrag zur Psychologie und Psychopathologie der Gestaltung*. Berlin: Springer; 1922.
2. Mello L. *Nise da Silveira: caminhos de uma psiquiatra rebelde*. Rio de Janeiro: Automática Edições; 2014.
3. Da Silveira N. *O mundo das imagens*. São Paulo: Ática; 1992.
4. Da Silveira N. *Casa das Palmeiras. A emoção de lidar. Uma experiência em psiquiatria*. Rio de Janeiro: Alhambra; 1986.
5. Priebe S, Omer S, Giacco D, et al. Resource-oriented therapeutic models in psychiatry: conceptual review. Br J Psychiatry. 2014;204:256–61. https://doi.org/10.1192/bjp.bp.113.135038.
6. Crawford J, Killaspy H, Barnes TRE, et al. Group art therapy as an adjunctive treatment for people with schizophrenia: multicentre pragmatic randomised trial. Brit Med J. 2012;344:e846. https://doi.org/10.1136/bmj.e846.

7. Bieleninik L, Geretsegger M, Mössler K, et al. Effects of improvisational music therapy vs enhanced standard care on symptom severity among children with autism spectrum disorder: The TIME-A randomised clinical trial. JAMA. 2017;318:525–35. https://doi.org/10.1001/jama.2017.9478.
8. Priebe S, Savill M, Wykes T, et al. Effectiveness of group body psychotherapy for negative symptoms of schizophrenia – a multi-centre randomised controlled trial. Br J Psychiatry. 2016;209:54–61. https://doi.org/10.1192/bjp.bp.115.171397.
9. Priebe S. A social paradigm in psychiatry – themes and perspectives. Epidemiol Psychiatr Sci. 2016;21:521–7. https://doi.org/10.1017/S2045796016000147.

Contents

Part I

Visual Art Therapy

Visual Art Therapy in Psychiatry Rehabilitation

1

Caterina Viganò and Roberta Magnotti

1.1 Introduction

Visual art therapies are a group of therapeutic techniques that use different creative and artistic media (such as drawing, painting, collage, colouring, and sculpting) "as its primary mode of expression and communication" [1] aiming to a global approach to the person. They refer to the person involving different communication channels (sensorial, cognitive, pragmatic, imaginative, intuitive, etc.) and expressive skills (verbal, non-verbal, artistic) in order to enhance the individual in its entirety. Within the expressive approach, the mental disorder is mainly seen as an alteration of the subject's relationship skills with himself and others. This inability to enter into and maintain valid object relations, in turn, reinforces the alteration of the capacity for thought and communication with the outside world. This kind of intervention is basically aimed at the most effective possible reconstitution of a functional organization of the structures of the intrapsychic self (bodily, expressive, verbal), which lie at the basis of object relation. The theme of creative expressions in their connection with the care processes constitutes an "open field with mobile boundaries" as Gillo Dorfles and Giorgio Bedoni discuss in a conversation on art and psychiatry [2]. Curing and caring in psychiatry emphasize the conceptual integration of therapy and rehabilitation: "it invests the whole person and the relationship with the therapist in a diadic fashion that evolves and constantly modifies" [3]. This happens

C. Viganò (✉)
Department of Biomedical and Clinical Sciences "Luigi Sacco", Università degli Studi di Milano, Milan, Italy

Psychiatric Rehabilitative Centres Unit, Second Psychiatric Unit, ASST Fatebenefratelli Sacco, Milan, Italy
e-mail: caterina.vigano@unimi.it

R. Magnotti
Psychiatric Rehabilitative Centres Unit, Second Psychiatric Unit, ASST Fatebenefratelli Sacco, Milan, Italy

U. Volpe (ed.), *Arts Therapies in Psychiatric Rehabilitation*,
https://doi.org/10.1007/978-3-030-76208-7_1

through the meeting of the individual resources of the two subjects, through mutual recognition. It is evident that such concepts are essential in a psychiatric context, where pain does not have an adequate mental representation, as we are accustomed to think mostly in verbal terms and the willingness to a human interaction is mainly based on verbal coding.

For the achievement of a positive result of care fundamental value is attributed to the model of "object relationships" [4] which emphasizes the process of internalization of the relationship with the therapist. Every person has a tendency to prefer a specific sensory channel (i.e., visual, auditory, cenesthetic) which can become predominant as an alternative to the usual ways in which thought evolves. An organic injury, as well as a psychic problem of any origin, can cause a sort of impediment of the normal transition from emotional experience to mentalization-symbolization and subsequent verbal expression of thought developed. In cases where the impediment has occurred to the transmission of one's emotional experience to the word, it may happen that the preferential sensory channel (channel becomes such preferential for a contest of experiences that have invested it with an imprinting of pleasant) of the subject is the only to allow the exchange at the level [5]. Such a complex of emotional experiences constitute that basic element, that unique "quid," subjective and specific for every individual, whose awareness can only be achieved through a relationship with another individual who has similar resources, but also technical knowledge. This specific communicative competence can be recognized, valued, and used through a process of reflection. Expressive therapies occupy this specific relational space created by whenever a trained practitioner discovers in a patient the presence of a curative potential that has to do with one of the artistic expressive channels (painting, dance, theatre, music, etc.) and gets in touch—or rather in relationship—with the client through a language within the transitional space [6]. In this sense, a crucial difference that needs to be pointed out is that between therapy and rehabilitation in psychiatry, as the two approaches often intertwine to each other but remain distinct with respect to main goals (even if both treatments globally aim at promoting personal change). In rehabilitation, the acquisition or recovery of skills, the enhancement of present resources, therefore a work on the subject's external, leads to a consequent internal rearrangement. In psychotherapy, the work involves the reassembly of the deeper, internal structures, with the consequent reorganization that is then shown at the external level [7]. A therapeutic relationship is managed in the clinical setting according to diverse techniques emanated from different theories. The Bionian theory [6] is combined with expressive therapies because it gives ample space to creative thought and emphasizes how the profound change takes form gradually without apparent common thread if not what there is between the two unconscious subjects in play and without a default target, but which is specified over time.

In the rehabilitation intervention, conversely, the sense of the relationship and the objectives of rehabilitation are defined from the beginning. It is therefore evident that therapy can be structured within rehabilitation, in a program that provides for their harmonious intertwining. In psychiatry, we art therapy is often intended as a rehabilitative therapeutic intervention that takes place through the free expression of one's creativity. Graphic production, through the activation of non-verbal communication, can replace the word as a means of communication and in psychotic patients in particular can represent an essential element of the therapeutic relationship [8]. By graphically expressing something that is unconsciously and consciously impossible to speak of, a first attempt is made to structure affective and emotional contents that are often chaotic, invasive, or even removed. To express oneself with art means not only to communicate something of oneself, but also to learn how to do it, modulating the instincts, the emotions as well as the thought.

In the last few decades, the concept of "Art Therapy" has been developed and reshaped in many different ways and has often been associated with various expressions such as "Creative Art Therapies" or "Expressive Therapies."

Following the definition given by the British Association of Art Therapists, Art Therapy is a "form of psychotherapy that uses graphic-pictorial artistic means, but not only, as a primary mode of communication" ([9]; www.baat.org). This definition, however, favors a conceptualization of art therapy meant as "art in therapy" (art represents an expressive and emotionally immediate means to be placed within a more structured psychotherapeutic path), with respect to the conceptualization known as "art as therapy" (that is, art as a form of re-socializing therapy and that eases emotional expression itself), doubtful for many, but still widely represented in the context of psychiatric rehabilitation [10]. Such a didactic distinction into two separate concepts of art therapy has often been criticized by artists who usually work in ateliers with psychiatric patients, as they often defend the internal and exclusive value of artistic expression as therapy, as a stimulus to creativity and well-being change also for patients with severe disorders, giving greater importance to the aesthetic value of the product rather than to the therapeutic value of the relationship [2].

1.2 History

In several countries, visual art therapy has experienced a substantially "bimodal spread" along the past century [11]: an initial professional interest in the use of the arts in psychiatry was expressed already in the first years of the twentieth century and had substantially followed, in the context of psychiatric hospitals, the international orientation ruled by the current psychoanalytic thought [12, 13].

Art therapy originated from the so-called *Psychopathology of Expression*, which saw in the graphic and artistic production of the mentally ill the representation of its pathology. In the second half of the nineteenth century, the interest in the figurative productions of the psychiatric patients inspired some nosographic and diagnostic research. Cesare Lombroso, in the second half of the nineteenth century, proposed that madness develops creativity, leaving the rest of the imagination free and therefore giving rise to creations that a too rational mind would not be able to produce, being more defended in the face of what is apparently illogical or absurd; he had long studied the correlation between genius and madness through the artistic productions of patients called "*art of the insane*" [14]. Also Max Simon [15] had given clinical diagnostic significance to the drawings of patients. Although this approach was disconfirmed in the twentieth century, it inspired the work of Hans Prinzhorn [16] who collected the drawings of "schizophrenic masters" (Heidelberg Collection) in the Heidelberg psychiatric clinic and first defined the creative drive as a "need for expression." He also differentiated primitive art, child art and that of the sick (alienated art) and began to question the diagnostic interest in the works of the sick, coming to the conclusion that the pictorial work is the expression and the manifestation of the personality of those who produced it in its entirety and cannot be considered only products of the disease or health of its author. Subsequently, the studies of Volmat [17] came to qualify the artistic activity as a possible historical testimony of the evolution of the pathological process.

Studies on the works of ill artists have shown that sometimes it is possible to witness the dissolution of personality by maintaining talent, while registering a change in style. This field of study is still active [18–20].

To achieve a proper analysis of the narrative value of the drawing, however, it was necessary to wait for an integration between the consideration of the artistic moment as objectification of the symptomatology and the interest oriented to the psychological history of the subject in terms of conflicts, defenses, and unconscious world. Mainly due to the psychoanalytic contributions, drawing began to be understood as a detector of unconscious instances and of the relational universe of the subject. Also at the beginning of the twentieth century, Jean Dubuffet, founder of the Compagnie de l'Art Brut in 1924, had observed that the artistic productions of mentally ill people often had aesthetic characteristics that combined them with some of the most interesting experiences of contemporary art. We recall here, as an example, the production of Carlo and Aloyse exhibited at the Art Brut Museum in Lausanne [21, 22].

In Europe, after the Second World War, a proliferation of art therapy ateliers with therapeutic purposes was established, with a predominance of the psychodynamic theoretical bases. The First International Psychopathological Art Exhibition, in Paris (1950), marked a turning point in this discipline. Robert Volmat's [17] volume "L'Art Psychopathologique" appeared in 1956 and in 1959 Volmat founded the International Society of Psychopathology of Expression. Also in the USA, about in the same period, there was an intense production on the subject. In the second half of the twentieth century, the texts on Art Therapy by Margaret Naumburg, Edith Kramer, Loretta Bender, and Paul Childer were published and the debate on its definition of art therapy was settled in the USA (art "in" therapy vs. art "as" therapy) [23].

Margaret Naumburg (1890–1983) focused her theory on the concept of art in therapy, seeing art as an instrument of a particular form of psychotherapy; she placed no emphasis on the aesthetic product in itself but on the communication process, which sees in artistic production a symbolic medium of the therapeutic relationship [24, 25]. Naumburg's deemphasis on the art product reflected her concept that *locus of change* in therapy was innate to the patient/art/therapist relationship and in the patient's increasing ability to use their art as mirror for self-understanding. Within the Naumburg framework, words played a very important part as they do in traditional psychoanalysis and psychotherapy [23]

Edith Kramer (1916–2014) instead conceptualized that the creative process in itself (art as therapy) was therapeutic which is very popular even today. She did not call herself a psychotherapist but a psychologically trained art teacher; she called his "clients" students: *"the art therapist ... communicates with his students via the students' painting and this communications has therapeutic value ... but he is no psychotherapist"* [26]. The main goal of her art therapy model was "personality change and healing through the vicissitudes of the creative process," she based her theory on Freudian development theories and saw art as a means of strengthening the ego, making sense of identity and encourage the maturation of the individual. Despite a good knowledge of analytical theories, she never used interpretation in working with children and gave the therapist an indication to use her psychoanalytic knowledge to help the child in the artistic expression of the emotional material [27]. Within this conceptual framework, the art therapist helps the patient (client) by providing them with artistic skills to facilitate the development of their creativity; above all, she did not consider the use of words during the session as crucial, defining the art studio (atelier) as a kind of "sanctuary," where a discussion was possible only after the work was finished and after putting everything in order [28].

The first trade magazine was the Bulletin of Art Therapy in 1962 and the American Art Therapy Association gathered for the first time in 1969. Various training programs were developed in the USA including master courses, in an attempt to give structured training to a discipline that was spreading as a credible mental health discipline. The 1970s witnessed the publication of the experiences of several art therapists, mainly as narrative clinical cases accompanied by images (as in the experiences of Lucille Venture, Georgette Seabrook Powell, and Cliff Joseph; see, [23]).

In the 1980s, the term *expressive arts therapy* appears as an integration of the main artistic techniques in the healing process and a university course focusing on this specific subject was also activated (Certificate Program in Expressive Therapies, at the Saybrook Graduate School and Research Center, San Francisco, CA). Three areas of study converge in this approach: the theory of object relations in art therapy, the "person-centered expressive art therapy," and a more shamanic vision of art therapy by Shaun McNiff.

The theory of object relations in art therapy used by A. Robbins may be defined as follows: "art therapy, then, strives to promote new levels of perceptual organization that involves shifts in energy patterns. The art form offers and added means for working with splits and polarities and integrating them into new wholes. The representations from our past are expressed through image and expand the boundaries of objective reality. " [29].

Shaun McNiff's theoretical conceptualization of the art therapist as shaman is unique in the history: he focused on socially applications of the technique and placed himself outside the medical model and within humanistic and transpersonal frame. His trans-cultural and anthropological approach was in contrast to most art therapist because his vision included an emphasis on spirituality and he argued that more Freudian based art therapist who struggle with making the unconscious conscious in their clients, still believed "in the will and the life spirit inside of and between the people" [30].

Natalie Rogers developed the person-centered expressive art therapy, believing that therapy and creativity overlap and goal of her work was "awaken the creative life force energy" [31]; she often worked with groups and her intention is to integrate the arts to help clients acting out deep inner conflicts facilitating their to resolution and healing [32].

Over the years, various American and British art therapy realities appeared and, in 1989, representatives from a dozen of countries met at the annual meeting of the Art Therapy Association (www.arttherapy.org) with the aim of creating an international network of art therapists (International networking group of Art Therapists, ING/AT). The ING/AT gathered more than 15,000 art therapists in 90 countries and, at the beginning of the twenty-first century, merged with the American Art Therapy Association (AATA).

In Great Britain, the use of art therapy as a healing technique had an increasing value in medical and psychiatric settings in the second half of the twentieth century and the art therapist was officially recognized as an assistant profession by the UK Health Profession Council in 1999. Many other European countries followed a similar evolution: for example, the Italian Art Therapy Society was founded in the 1980s, deriving some professional core concepts from the art-therapist figure as defined by the British Association Art Therapy. What emerges from several authors is that giving common meaning to art therapy is difficult even within the same nation; there are many approaches, as diversified training schools have been created over the years. The debate remains open on the definition of the criteria for a curing technique to be defined as art therapy, such as the requirements and skills that art therapists must have and what is meant by training to improve the scientific relevance of this technique [33].

Finally, in recent times thanks to a more and more active dialogue between art and neuroscience, we can introduce a period of renewed research in the history of art therapy. Recent evidence-based developments in neurobiology have made it possible to see art therapy as a mind/body practice that provides a means of regulation through the cognitive and sensorial processing. The artistic experience may favor neural plasticity, in terms of peripheral stimulation of the different sensory modalities, spontaneous expression of the emotions, complex cognitive activities (involving internal decisions and images) and motor activity [34].

Neurological studies confirm how art therapy can rebalance brain functions that have been compromised by trauma and other emotional connection losses [35, 36]. Recent brain imaging studies, using advanced technologies (such as fMRI) reveal information about how a person process stimuli that cannot otherwise be observed or self-reported, highlighted how art therapy is able to promote cognitive and sensory processing of experiences, favoring emotional regulation. In particular, some studies showed arts' beneficial effects in cases of stress-related trauma: through art, in a therapeutic context, it is possible to give expression to what cannot be expressed in words, find containment for the experience and ease its processing [37].

Over the last decades of the twentieth century, different art-therapeutic approaches have spread in Europe and in the USA, based on empirical evidence (although not systematically collected and sometimes methodologically flawed) demonstrating a good impact on resocialization processes at reasonable costs. However, with the critical review of psychoanalytic paradigms and the shift towards community-oriented psychiatry paradigms, in the second half of the twentieth century, art therapy was often associated with an indiscriminate and, sometimes, inappropriate application of the abovementioned techniques, which have probably led to a drift dragging these approaches, like other rehabilitative ones, increasingly towards entertainment and away from proper psychiatric rehabilitation practice [7, 38–40].

With the transition into the third millennium, the use of art in psychiatric rehabilitation has experienced a new impulse associated with greater methodological rigor and the accumulation of growing scientific evidence. Several randomized controlled trials, focusing on art therapy, have been conducted over the last decades and have demonstrated, with a greater methodological rigor and standardized outcomes measures, the effectiveness of such rehabilitative approaches as an additional treatment in different mental and neurological disorders [41–51].

Another general characteristic of this "second wave" of studies focusing on the application of artistic techniques to psychiatric rehabilitation was that of the application of different conceptual reference models (beyond the classical psychoanalytic framework and including cognitive, narrative, systemic-relational, patient-centered orientations) in different target populations: while in the past most of the programs were performed for patients with chronic psychoses in rehabilitation centers, recently patients with various psychiatric diagnoses, often with a recent history of illness and different levels of severity, have been involved in artistic rehabilitation programs in different settings (i.e., territorial psychiatric facilities and rehabilitation residences), in both short- and long-term programs, as reported in several critical reviews and meta-analysis [51–54].

Overall, in the last decade some evidences of the effectiveness of visual art therapy on specific psychological and symptomatological dimensions and in different age groups are appearing, even if a general agreement in the field does not exist yet [55].

Given the increasing availability of more reliable scientific evidence on the implementation of art therapy programs in psychiatry, it is not surprising that such techniques have been included in guidelines for treatment of mental illnesses. So far, the National Collaborating Center for Mental Health [56] included art therapies among the recommended treatment "to promote, with pharmacotherapy and structured psychotherapy, the healing of patients with schizophrenia, especially if young and with prevalent affective and/or negative symptoms." Although the evidence from randomized controlled trials is limited at the present moment [57], art therapy is very much used in psychiatric rehabilitation settings and empirical evidence that favors its use in psychiatry is accumulating over the past years [52]. Small numbers of patients reported varying reasons for not wanting to take part, and some highlighted potentially negative effects of art therapy which included the evoking of feelings which could not be resolved. The findings suggest that for the majority of respondents art therapy was an acceptable intervention, although this was not the case for all respondents. Therefore, attention should be focused on both identifying those who are most likely to benefit from art therapy and ensuring any potential harms are minimized [58].

Beyond the debate on effectiveness of art therapies in the real-world psychiatric settings, another aspect warranted more and more attention within the field, relating to the mechanisms of change related to the application of art-therapeutic approaches.

1.3 Basic Principles and Techniques

Recently, Dunphy et al. [43] proposed a classification of the main mechanisms for change for negative and depressive symptoms through art interventions, which are reported in Table 1.1.

Visual art methods include various types of painting and drawing (clay work, sculpting, collage, mask making), materials (watercolors, wax pencil, color pencil, acrylic colors, etc.) and techniques can be selected or focused on specific populations (children, adults) or diagnosis (trauma, psychotic disorders, addictions) [72].

In a rehabilitation program art therapists often recommend during first sessions free theme drawing, or gestural; for suspicious patients at the beginning may be useful geometrical figures. Simplify mandala is a good suggestion for frozen psychotic patient. Human body drawings, portrait, body tracing and other techniques need a stronger therapeutical relationship [73].

Table 1.1 Basic principles of visual art therapy

Physical effects	Engagement in a creative activity that had physical aspects was seen to catalyze relaxation and reduction of stress [59–62]
Cultural effects	Making of art was seen to facilitate creative expression and play [46, 63]; creative expression was enabled by use of accessible media of clay and painting [60]; evocation of familiarity and positive memories was catalyzed by use of culturally appropriate traditional crafts and arts [41, 63]
Emotional/ intrapersonal effects	Creation of art products was seen to: (a) provide valuable distance and enable externalization and visual communication of inner subjective experiences [41, 60, 61, 64–68]; (b) facilitate expression of positive and negative emotions [46, 64, 67–69]; (c) promote the development of autonomy [59, 60, 69–71]; (d) stimulate self esteem [41, 49, 59, 63, 65, 69] and agency [41, 45, 62, 63, 70]
Cognitive effects	Reinforcement and recall of positive memories [45, 46, 59, 66] and distraction from ruminative thoughts [41, 60]
Interpersonal effects	Group work, with or without therapist's involvement, was seen to encourage socialization and sharing [46, 49, 59, 62, 63, 65–69, 71]

1.4 Available Evidence

A bibliographic database search on Pubmed and other scientific literature databases revealed more than 10,000 papers, the first one published in the journal *l'Encephale* by Bergeron and Volmat [74] although a specific role of art as a therapeutic approach in Psychiatry is recognized with scientific evidence only by the end of the twentieth century [16, 24, 25, 28, 42, 54, 66, 75–77]. Below is provided a synthesis of the available evidence on the use of visual art therapy in psychiatric rehabilitation, according to specific groups of disorders.

1.4.1 Psychotic Disorders

Many studies have been published during last decades, as Chaing et al. [78] extensively describe, but the first randomized controlled study on visual art therapy for schizophrenia was carried out by an English group [79]. The Matisse Project Team did not report an advantage of the add-on of art therapy to standard treatments delivered to patients with schizophrenia, with respect to global functioning and clinical outcomes. The negative view associated to this evidence could be partially tempered by considering that the chosen outcome indicators may represent an extensive measure that might not be suitable to capture properly the peculiarity of the change processes activated by expressive therapy. Several studies have then appeared in literature with the aim of analyzing the therapeutic effect of art therapy for schizophrenic patients, but with a less quantitative approach and using standard clinical dimensions as indicators. Overall, many studies have demonstrated that art therapy may reduce the levels of negative symptoms in schizophrenia [80] but also improve self-knowledge, interpersonal skills, and affective development, at least at the same level of other psychosocial interventions conducted among psychotic patients [53]. For example, a study conducted in the United Kingdom on acute psychiatric inpatients [81] has stressed that participation in structured sessions of art therapy can change the subjective experience in a positive sense and restore a sense of hope in the future, increase participants' level of emotional awareness and ability to reflect on other people's emotional states, thus indirectly acting on positive affective dimensions and recovery. Another study conducted in Norway [82] reported very similar results, observing an improvement in the insight and management of positive symptoms of schizophrenia (especially if art therapy is embedded into structured treatment programs). Later on, Attard and Larkin [52] published a review of the literature on the effectiveness of art therapy for psychotic patients, in which they examined 18 high-quality quantitative studies on art therapy in schizophrenia, but authors concluded that valid studies are still a small number in literature and thus scientific evidence of the efficacy of art therapy in adults with psychosis has still to be considered inconclusive.

A limitation inherent to the randomized clinical trial aimed at measuring the effectiveness of art therapy in psychotic patients is the use of standard symptom outcome indicators, mostly positive and negative symptoms [83], while it would probably be more appropriate to use extensive indicators that also take into account qualitative and subjective dimensions, as well as emotional experiences.

In a study conducted on patients dwelling in community facilities (i.e., psychiatric rehabilitation community and day center) for whom the "Optimal Experience" approach was adopted, Bassi et al. [84] examined with the experience sampling method a state characterized by the perception of high challenges and high skills, deep concentration, positive affect, clear goals, control and autonomous motivation, which contributes to individuals' well-being. Authors reported that the "flow" state was most evident when patients were engaged in rehabilitation activities, particularly during art therapy sessions (while it did not occur during non-structured activities or leisure time).

A possible limit in the design of randomized controlled studies conducted to evaluate art therapy programs may lie in the patient's level of motivation towards the activity, a condition that enables a constant adherence to the activity [85]: although motivation and engagement may be crucial to produce optimal results with art therapy approaches, they are not systematically measured in scientific studies within this field [86].

However, there are some qualitative studies in the literature which show art therapy can be used as a significant, acceptable and advantaged intervention in psychotic disorders, although this conclusion is based on a small number of studies [52].

1.4.2 Affective Disorders

Art therapy programs are often delivered to patients with affective disorders of all ages [87], although most of published studies in the international literature on art therapy and depression actually concern the elderly population [62, 78]. For some people, art therapy may be a more acceptable alternative form of psychological therapy than standard forms of treatment, such as talking therapies [51]. Dunphy et al. [43] recently confirmed that the use of artistic techniques in this population induce improvement of mood and physical state, more connected to the techniques like dance movement therapy and dramatherapy but more generally of the subjective perception of well-being and enhanced self-concept, of the processes of elaboration of the emotions, of the cognitive functions like memory [41, 87, 88]. Viégas Brandão et al. [89] also reported that manual work (drawing, painting, and modeling) and contemplation of art pieces are most represented and that most of the researches are European in this field of work. While the most recent edition of the UK guidelines for depression in adolescents suggest the use of art therapies [90], less data are available on subjects in the 14–18 age group and also in these studies the indicators of outcome are mostly quantitative (mostly a reduction in symptomatology) and effects on positive affective dimensions are rarely considered. However, in a recent controlled study on such population [91], participation in just six art therapy sessions improved the dimension of *internalization*, which is often linked to depressive/anxious symptoms and withdrawal, thus providing a more solid theoretical basis for the use of these techniques in adolescents with anxiety, depression, and withdrawal disorders.

1.4.3 Anxiety and Post-Traumatic Disorders

In clinical practice, art therapy is often provided as an additional therapy to patients with anxiety disorders and PTSD [92–96] but currently there is no evidence of effectiveness of AT on the reduction of anxiety symptoms and no overview of intervention characteristics. Some of available reviews are focused on treatment included art therapy in a broader definition of psychodynamic therapies [97]. In a recent systematic review of 776 publications, Abbing et al. [98] find that art therapy is possibly effective in reducing pre-exam anxiety in students and pre-release anxiety in prisoners. Authors hyphothesized working mechanism of art therapy as inducing relaxation, gaining access to unconscious traumatic memories [99–101], thereby creating possiblities to investigate cognitions and improve emotional regulation [102].

1.4.4 Eating Disorders

Art-based interventions are increasingly being employed as adjunctive treatments for eating disorders (anorexia nervosa and binge eating disorders) to help patients express and explore emotions [103] but it has not seen systematically studied [104–107] and art therapy is not referenced in most recent guidelines [108].

1.4.5 Others Neuropsychiatric Disorders

Historically drawing and painting have been recognized as a useful part of therapeutic processes within medical and neurology based disciplines [109]. Art-based therapies are generally considered as low cost and useful interventions to improve well-being and quality of life in older people [88], not only depressed, and it's used for managing manifestations of dementia in earlier stages, as they may help to slow cognitive deterioration, address symptoms related to psychosocial challenging behaviors, and improve quality of life [48, 64, 110], but a recent Cochrane review [111] concludes there is insufficient evidence from randomized controlled trials to draw any reliable conclusions about efficacy of art therapy on cognition, affect and emotional well-being and social functioning for people with dementia and there is a clear need for more RTC addressed to reduce methodological bias.

1.5 Future Directions

Already some years ago, Reynolds et al. [112] pointed out that the body of knowledge in the field of art therapy in psychiatry was significantly grown and established itself significantly, as witnessed by the increasing number of randomized controlled trials (with level 1 scientific evidence) conducted with larger sample sizes on this topic. The advantage of such studies lies in the lesser likelihood of Type I errors as opposed to other studies with no control group or studies that have a control group but no randomization. Nevertheless, there are still only a small number of studies addressing each population, and these studies differ considerably in terms of the course of the therapeutic process, the proposed interventions, and the indices that were examined. Although the possibility to make direct comparisons among studies in this area of research is difficult, a general trend towards the global increase of the quality of studies focusing on art therapy, with more carefully study designs, can be traced and this may ease the processes of validation and replication of studies in the future. Therefore taking into account all these aspects, new development of research will be set in the future in this field. They would consider a better characterization of patients (age, gender, diagnosis, cognitive functioning, staging of illness, therapies), test larger sample is needed, but first of all it's necessary to establish what outcomes, what dimensions are to be assessed, and what psychometrics instruments, in a rehabilitative psychiatric setting.

To conclude, it's necessary to point out that art therapy is a set of techniques that cannot be improvised and it requires specialized training to be applied. Despite the need for trained personnel, it seems that in the studies on the costs of the different interventions, art therapy does not seem more expensive than other ones, as highlighted by the PROSPERO study for the National Institute for Health Research Health Technology Assessment [113] where he states that art therapy was associated with positive effects when compared with a control in a number of studies in patients with different clinical profiles, and it was reported to be an acceptable treatment and was associated with a number of benefits. Art therapy appeared to be cost-effective compared with wait-list but further studies are needed to confirm this finding as well as evidence to inform future cost-effective analyses of art therapy versus other treatments.

References

1. British Association of Art Therapists. About art therapy. 2019. https://www.baat.org. Accessed Jan 2019.
2. Bedoni G, Tosatti L. Arte e psichiatria. In: Uno sguardo sottile. Milano: Mazzotta; 2000.
3. Palazzi Trivelli C. Artiterapie, i fondamenti. Torino: Tirrenia Stampatori; 2000.
4. Hughes JM. In: Fairbairn WRD, Winnicott DW, editors. Reshaping the psychoanalytic domain. the work of Melanie Klein. 1st ed. CA: California University Press; 1989.
5. Pistorio G. Arte e psichiatria. In: Palazzi Trivelli C, editor. Artiterapie, i fondamenti. Torino: Tirrenia Stampatori; 2000.

6. Bion WR. Learning from experience. London: William Heinemann; 1962. (Reprinted London: Karnac Books) (trad. it.: Apprendere dall'esperienza, Roma: Armando, 1972).
7. Ba G. Strumenti e tecniche di riabilitazione psichiatrica e psicosociale. Milano: FrancoAngeli; 2003.
8. Czamanski-Cohen J, Weihs KL. The bodymind model: a platform for studying the mechanisms of change induced by art therapy. Arts Psychother. 2016;51:63–71. https://doi.org/10.1016/j.aip.2016.08.006.
9. Waller D. Becoming a profession: a history of art therapy 1940–82. London: Routledge; 1991.
10. Edwards D. Art therapy. London: Sage; 2004.
11. Volpe U, Facchini D, Magnotti R, Diamare S, Denti E, Viganò CA. Le arti-terapie nel contesto della riabilitazione psicosociale italiana: una rassegna critica. Psichiatria Psicoterapia. 2016;35(4):154–80.
12. Freeman RD, Friedman I. Art therapy in a total treatment plan. J Nerv Ment Dis. 1956;124(4):421–5.
13. Killick K. Art therapy for psychosis. Theory and practice. NY: Routlegde; 2017.
14. Lombroso C. The man of genius. London: Walter Scott; 1891.
15. Max S. Le ecrits et le dessins des alienes. Lyon: Arch. Anthrop. Crim; 1888.
16. Prinzhorn H. Bildnerei der Geisteskranken. Ein Beitrag zur Psychologie und Psychopatologie der Gestaltung – artistry of the mentally ill: a contribution to the psychology and psychopathology of configuration. Translated by Eric von Brockdorff from the second German edition, with an introduction by James L. Foy. 1995. Wien, New York: Springer-Verlag; 1922.
17. Volmat R. L'Art Psychopathologique. Paris: PUF; 1956.
18. Leipzig BE, Minkowska F. De van Gogh et Searux aux dessins d'enfants. Paris: Presses du temps present; 1949.
19. Jakab I. The history of the founding of societe de psychopathologie de l'expression and early development. Psychiatr Hung. 2010;25(4):276–90.
20. van Emmerik Arnold AP, Hamaker EL. Paint it black: using change-point analysis to investigate increasing vulnerability to depression towards the end of Vincent van Gogh's life. Healthcare. 2017;5:53. https://doi.org/10.3390/healthcare5030053.
21. Andreoli V. The graphic language of madness. Milan: Masson; 1982.
22. Porret-Forel J. Aloyse ou la peinture magique d'une schizophrene. These Medical Lausanne; 1958.
23. Borowsky Junge M. The modern history of art therapy in the United States. Springfield, IL: Charles C. Thomas Publisher Ltd; 2010.
24. Naumburg M. Psychoneurotic art: its function in psychotherapy. New York: Grune & Stratton; 1953.
25. Naumburg M. Dynamically oriented art therapy. Its principles and practice, illustrated with three case studies. New York: Grune & Stratton; 1966.
26. Kramer E. Art therapy in children's community. NY: Charles C. Thomas; 1958.
27. Kramer E. Art as therapy with children. NY: Schocken; 1971.
28. Kramer E. Art as therapy: collected papers. London: Jessica Kingsley Publishers; 2000.
29. Robbins A. Object relations art therapy. In: Rubin J, editor. Approaches to art therapy. NY: Brunner/Mazel; 1987.
30. McNiff S. The art in psychotherapy. Springfield, IL: Charles C. Thomas; 1981.
31. Rubin AJ. Approaches to art therapy: theory and techniques. 2nd ed. New York: Routlegde; 2001.
32. Roger N. The creative connection: expressive arts as healing. Palo Alto, CA: Science and Behavior Books; 1993.
33. Della Cagnoletta M. Art therapy the psychodynamic perspective. Roma: Carocci; 2010.
34. Lusenbrick VB. Imagery and visual expresión in therapy. Nueva Cork: Plenum; 1994.
35. Garner RL. The Nat model: factors in neuropsychological art therapy. Am J Art Ther. 1996;34:107–11.
36. McNamee CM. Bilateral art: integrating art therapy, family therapy, and neuroscience. Contemp Fam Ther. 2005;27:545. https://doi.org/10.1007/s10591-005-8241-y.

37. Noah H-C, Carr M. Art therapy and clinical neuroscience. London: Jessica Kingsley Publishers; 2008.
38. Ba G, Viganò C. L'arte terapia nel percorso riabilitativo del paziente psicotico. In: Quaderni di Castel Ivano: "La riabilitazione in Psichiatria". Strigno Trento: LitoDelta; 1996. p. 32–4.
39. Ba G, Magnotti R, Olivani F, Vigano C. Le tecniche espressive in riabilitazione psichiatrica. In: Bellazzecca C, Peserico M, Rabboni M, editors. Curare con le arti. Neuroscienze e tecniche espressive. Milano: Update International Congress; 2006. p. 43–50.
40. Saraceno B. La fine dell'intrattenimento. Manuale di riabilitazione psichiatrica. Milano: Etas; 1995.
41. Ciasca EC, Ferreira RC, Santana CLA, Forlenza OV, dos Santos GD, Brum PS, et al. Art therapy as an adjuvant treatment for depression in elderly women: a randomized controlled trial. Brazil J Psychiatry. 2018;40:256–63. https://doi.org/10.1590/1516-4446-2017-2250.
42. Crawford MJ, Patterson S. Arts therapies for people with schizophrenia: an emerging evidence base. Evid Based Mental Health. 2007;10(3):69–70.
43. Dunphy K, Baker FA, Dumaresq E, Carroll-Haskins K, Eickholt J, Ercole M, Kaimal G, Meyer K, Sajnani N, Shamir OY, Wosch T. Creative arts interventions to address depression in older adults: a systematic review of outcomes, processes, and mechanisms. Front Psychol. 2019;9:2655. https://doi.org/10.3389/fpsyg.2018.02655.
44. Hannemann BT. Creativity with dementia patients. Can creativity and art stimulate dementia patients positively? Gerontology. 2006;52(1):59–65.
45. Hoffmann NC. Using art therapy to address cognitive symptoms of Parkinson's disease. Int J User Driven Healthcare. 2013;3:74–95. https://doi.org/10.4018/ijudh.2013070106.
46. Kim HK, Kim KM, Nomura S. The effect of group art therapy on older Korean adults with neurocognitive disorders. Arts Psychother. 2016;47:48–54. https://doi.org/10.1016/j.aip.2015.11.002.
47. Koch S. Arts and health: active factors and a theory framework of embodied aesthetics. Arts Psychother. 2017;54:85–91. https://doi.org/10.1016/j.aip.2017.02.002.
48. Pongan E, Tillmann B, Leveque Y, Trombert B, Getenet JC, Auguste N, Dauphinot V, El Haouari H, Navez M, Dorey JM, Krolak-Salmon P, Laurent B, Rouch I, LACMé Group. Can musical or painting interventions improve chronic pain, mood, quality of life, and cognition in patients with mild Alzheimer's disease? Evidence from a randomized controlled trial. J Alzheimers Dis. 2017;60(2):663–77.
49. Rawtaer I, Mahendran R, Yu J, Fam J, Feng L, Kua EH. Psychosocial interventions with art, music, tai chi and mindfulness for subsyndromal depression and anxiety in older adults: a naturalistic study in Singapore. Asia Pac Psychiatry. 2015;7(3):240–50. https://doi.org/10.1111/appy.12201.
50. Sherwood P. Expressive artistic therapies as mind-body medicine. Body Mov Dance Psychother. 2008;3(2):81–95.
51. Uttley L, Scope A, Stevenson M, Rawdin A, Taylor Buck E, Sutton A, Stevens J, Kaltenthaler E, Dent-Brown K, Wood C. Systematic review and economic modelling of the clinical effectiveness and cost effectiveness of art therapy among people with non-psychotic mental health disorders. Health Technol Assess. 2015;19(18):1–120.
52. Attard A, Larkin M. Art therapy for people with psychosis: a narrative review of the literature. Lancet Psychiatry. 2016;3(11):1067–78.
53. De Silva MJ, Cooper S, Li HL, Lund C, Patel V. Effect of psychosocial interventions on social functioning in depression and schizophrenia: meta-analysis. Br J Psychiatry. 2013;202(4):253–60.
54. Regev D, Cohen-Yatziv L. Effectiveness of art therapy with adult clients in 2018—what progress has been made? Front Psychol. 2018;9:1531. https://doi.org/10.3389/fpsyg.2018.01531.
55. Viganò C, Wenk M, Ferrara L, Magnotti R, Borsani S. The "state of the Art" of art therapy in psychiatry: reflections on international evidences and Italian experiences. J. Complement Med Alter Healthcare. 2019;10(5):555796. https://doi.org/10.19080/JCMAH.2019.10.555796.

56. UK National Collaborating Centre for Mental Health. Schizophrenia: Core interventions in the treatment and management of schizophrenia in adults in primary and secondary care. London: The British Psychological Society and the Royal College of Psychiatrists; 2010.
57. Bastiampillai T, Allison S, Gupta A. NICE guidelines for schizophrenia: can art therapy be justified? Lancet Psychiatry. 2016;3(11):1016–7.
58. Scope A, Uttley L, Sutton A. A qualitative systematic review of service user and service provider perspectives on the acceptability, relative benefits and potential harms of art therapy for people with non psychotic mental health disorders. Psychol Psychother. 2017;90(1):25–43.
59. Canuto A, Meiler-Mitielu C, Herrmann FR, Delaloye C, Giannakopoulos P, Weber K. Longitudinal assessment of psychotherapeutic day hospital treatment for elderly patients with depression. Int J Geriatr Psychiatry. 2008;23:949–56. https://doi.org/10.1002/gps.2016.
60. Goldblatt R, Elkis-Abuhoff D, Gaydos M, Napoli A. Understanding clinical benefits of modeling clay exploration with patients diagnosed with Parkinson's disease. Arts Health. 2010;2:140–8. https://doi.org/10.1080/17533010903495405.
61. Hsu T-J, Tsai H-T, Hwang A-C, Chen L-Y, Chen L-K. Predictors of non-pharmacological intervention effect on cognitive function and behavioral and psychological symptoms of older people with dementia. Geriatr Gerontol. 2017;17:8–36. https://doi.org/10.1111/ggi.13037.
62. Hei L. Effectiveness of expressive arts therapy for elderly with depression and anxiety. Post graduate dissertation, University of Hong Kong;2015.
63. De Guzman AB, Satuito JCB, Satumba MAE, Segui DRA, Serquina FEC, Serrano LJP, et al. Filipino arts among elders in institutionalized care settings. Educ Gerontol. 2011;37:248–61. https://doi.org/10.1080/03601270903534937.
64. Kang H, Bae Y, Kim E, Lee K, Chae M, Ju R. An integrated dementia intervention for Korean older adults. J Psychosoc Nurs Ment Health Serv. 2010;48:42–50. https://doi.org/10.3928/02793695-20100930-01.
65. Draghici R. Experiential psychotherapy in geriatric groups. PRO. 2012;33:979–83. https://doi.org/10.1016/j.sbspro.2012.01.268.
66. Choi YH, Jeon EY. The effects of group art therapy on cognition, depression and quality of life in elderly. J Korean Acad Comm Health Nurs. 2013;24:323–31. https://doi.org/10.12799/jkachn.2013.24.3.323.
67. Ali K, Gammidge T, Waller D. Fight like a ferret: a novel approach of using art therapy to reduce anxiety in stroke patients undergoing hospital rehabilitation. Med Humanit. 2014;40:50–60. https://doi.org/10.1136/medhum-2013-010448.
68. Im ML, Lee JI. Effects of art and music therapy on depression and cognitive function of the elderly. Technol Health Care. 2014;22:453–8. https://doi.org/10.3233/THC-140803.
69. Kongkasuwan R, Voraakhom K, Pisolayabutra P, Maneechai P, Boonin J, Kuptniratsaikul V. Creative art therapy to enhance rehabilitation for stroke patients: a randomized controlled trial. Clin RehabIL. 2016;30:1016–23. https://doi.org/10.1177/0269215515607072.
70. Doric-Henry L. Pottery as art therapy with elderly nursing home residents. J Am Art Ther Assoc. 1997;14:163–71. https://doi.org/10.1080/07421656.1987.10759277.
71. Ceramidas DM. Faith-based cognitive behavioral therapy: easing depression in the elderly with cognitive decline. J Christ Nurs. 2012;29:42–8. https://doi.org/10.1097/CNJ.0b013e318238f288.
72. Potash JS, Ho RT, Chick JK, Au Yeung FS. Viewing and engaging in art therapy exhibit by people living with mental illness: implications for empathy and social change. Public Health. 2013;127(8):735–44.
73. Ba G. Metodologia della Riabilitazione psicosociale. Milano: FrancoAngeli; 1994. p. 315–50.
74. Bergeron M, Volmat R. Collective art in mental disorders. Encéphale. 1952;41(2):143–211.
75. Hill A. Art versus illness: a story of art therapy. London: Allen & Unwin; 1945.
76. MacGregor JM. The discovery of the art of the insane. Princeton: Princeton University Press; 1989.
77. Schneider Adams L. Art and psychoanalysis. New York: Harper Collins; 1993.
78. Chaing M, Reid-Varley WB, Fan X. Creative art therapy for mental illness. Psychiatr Res. 2019;275:129–36. https://doi.org/10.1016/j.psychres.2019.03.025.

79. Crawford MJ, Killapsy H, Kalaitzaki E, Barrett B, Byford S, Patterson S, Soteriosu T, O'Neill F, Clayton K, Maratos A, Barnes RT, Osborn D, Johson T, King M, Tyrer P, Waller D. The MATISSE study: a randomised trial of group art therapy for people with schizophrenia. BMC Psychiatry. 2010;10:65.
80. Lutgens D, Gariepy G, Malla A. Psychological and psychosocial interventions for negative symptoms in psychosis: systematic review and meta-analysis. Br J Psychiatry. 2017;210(5):324–32.
81. Sticley T, Hui A. Arts in-reach: taking bricks off shoulders in adult mental health inpatient care. J Psychiatr Ment Health Nurs. 2012;19(5):402–9.
82. Hanevik H, Hestad K, Lien L, Stube Teglbjaerg H, Danbolt LH. Expressive art therapy for psychosis: a multiple case study. Arts Psychother. 2013;40(3):312–21.
83. Montag C, Haase L, Seidel D, Bayerl M, Gallinat J, Herrmann U, Dannecker K. A pilot RCT of psychodynamic group art therapy for patients in acute psychotic episodes: feasibility, impact on symptoms and mentalising capacity. PLoS One. 2014;9(11):e112348.
84. Bassi M, Ferrario N, Ba G, Delle Fave A, Viganò C. Quality of experience during psychosocial rehabilitation: a real time investigation with experience sampling method. Psychiatr Rehabil J. 2012;35(6):447–53.
85. Crawford M, Killaspy H, Barnes TR, Barrett B, Byford S, Clayton K, Dinsmore J, Floyd S, Hoadley A, Johnson T, Kalaitzaki E, King M, Leurent B, Maratos A, O'Neill FA, Osborn DP, Patterson S, Soteriou T, Tyrer P, Waller D, MATISSE Project Team. Group art therapy as adjunctive treatment for people with schizophrenia: multicentre pragmatic randomised trial. BMJ. 2012;344:*e846*.
86. Kurei-Chou, Shih YA-W, Chang C, Chou Y-Y, Hu W-H, Cheng J-S, Yang C-Y, Hsieh C-J. Psychosocial rehabilitation Activities, empowerment, and quality of community based life for people with schizophrenia. Arch Psychiatr Nurs. 2012;26(4):285–94.
87. Nan JKM, Ho RTH. Effects of clay art therapy on adults outpatients with major depressive disorder: a randomized controlled trial. J Affect Disord. 2017; https://doi.org/10.1016/j.jad.2017.04.013.
88. Roswiyani R, Kwakkenbos L, Spijker J, Witteman Cilia LM. The effectiveness of combining visual art activities and physical exercise for older adults on well being or quality of life and mood: a scoping review. J Appl Gerontol. 2019;38(12):1784–804.
89. Viégas Brandão FM, Ventura Silva C, da Silva Gonçalves de Oliveira KR, da Silva Pedroso J. Art as a therapeutic tool in depressive disorders: a systematic review of the literature. Psychiatr Q. 2019;90:871–82.
90. NICE Guidelines National Institute for health and care excellence. Depression in children and young people. 25 Sept 2019 online.
91. Bagarzan Y, Pakdaman S. The effectiveness of art therapy in reducing internalizing and externalizing problems of female adolescents. Arch Iran Med. 2016;19(1):51–6.
92. Hunter RS. Drawing soldiers out of post traumatic stress disorder. Mil Med Res. 2019;6(5) https://doi.org/10.1186/s40779-019-0195-8.
93. Nanda U, Barbato Gaydos HL, Hathom K, Watkins N. Art and post traumatic Stress: a review of the empirical literature on the therapeutic implications of artwork for war veterans with posttraumatic stress disorder. Environ Behav. 2010;42(3):376–90.
94. Ramirez JA. A review of art therapy among military service members and veterans with posttraumatic stress disorder. J Mil Veterans Health. 2016;24(2).
95. Schouten KA, de Niet GJ, Knipscheer JW, Kleber RJ, Hutschemaekers GJM. The effectiveness of art therapy in the treatment of traumatized adults. Trauma Violence Abuse. 2014;16(2):220–8.
96. Williams ME, Thompson SC. The use of community based interventions in reducing morbidity from the psychological impact of conflict related trauma among refugees population: a systematic review of literature. J Immigr Minor Health. 2010;13(4):780–94.
97. Fonagy P. The effectiveness of psychodynamic psychotherapies. An update. World Psychiatry. 2015;14(2):137–50.

98. Abbing A, Ponstein A, van Hooren S, de Sonneville L, Swaab H, Baar E. Effectiveness of art therapy for anxiety in adults: a systematic review of randomised and non-randomised controlled trials. PLOS One. 2018;13(12):e0208716.
99. Henderson P, Rosen D, Mascaro N. Empirical study on the healing nature of mandalas. Psychol Aesthet Creat Arts. 2007;24(2):71–5.
100. Sandimire DA, Gorham SR, Rankin NE, Grimm DR. The influence of art making on anxiety: a pilot study. Art Ther. 2012;29(2):68–73.
101. Yu YZ, Yu MC, Yue M, Hai Li J, Ling L. House-tree-person drawing therapy as an intervention for prisoners' prerelease anxiety. Soc Behav Pers. 2016;44(6):987–1004.
102. Drozdek B, Kamperman AM, Bolwerk N, Tol WA, Kleber RJ. Group therapy with male asylum seekers and refugees with post traumatic stress disorders. J Nerv Ment Dis. 2012;200(9):758–65.
103. Silverstone L. Art therapy exercises. London: Jessica Kingsley Publishers; 2009.
104. Frisch MJ, Franko DL, Herzog DB. Arts based therapies in the treatment of eating disorders. Eat Disord. 2006;14(2):131–42.
105. Garner DM, Rockert W, Davis R, Garner VM, Olmsted MP, Eagle W. Comparison of cognitive behavioural and supportive expressive therapy for bulimia nervosa. Am J Psychlatry. 1993;150(1):37–46.
106. Jarrige M, Calestreme M, Sudres JL. Art therapy in anorexia: the mediative elements? Soins Psychiatr. 2015;2015(298):40–4.
107. Lock J, Fitzpatrick KK, Agras WS, Weinbach N, Booil JO. Feasibility study combining art therapy or cognitive remediation therapy with family based treatment for adolescent anorexia nervosa. Eur Eat Disord Rev. 2018;26(1):62–8.
108. Couturier J, Isserlin L, Norris M, Spettigue W, et al. Canadian practice guidelines for the treatment of children and adolescent with eating disorders. J Eat Disorders. 2020;8:24. https://doi.org/10.1186/s40337-020-0277-8.
109. Flaherty AW. Brain illness and creativity: mechanims and treatment risks. Can J Psychiatry. 2011;56(3):132–43.
110. Burton A. Bringing arts based therapies in from the scientific cold. Lancet Neurol. 2009;8(9):784–5.
111. Deshmukh SR, Holmes J, Cardno A. Art therapy for people with dementia (review). Cochrane Database Syst Rev. 2018;(9):CD011073.
112. Reynolds MW, Nabors L, Quinlan A. The effectiveness of art therapy: does it work? Art Ther. 2000;17:207–13. https://doi.org/10.1080/07421656.2000.10129706.
113. Stevenson M, Scope A, Rawdin A, Sutton A. The clinical and cost effectiveness of group art therapy for people with non-psychotic mental health disorders: a systematic review and cost-effectiveness analysis. BMC Psychiatry. 2015;15:151. https://doi.org/10.1186/s12888-015-0528-4.

Between Subjectivity and Objectivity: Art Therapy's Challenge

2

Mimma Della Cagnoletta

As art therapists, we are always engaged in observing and thinking about our clients' artwork in order to understand their ways of expressing and communicating through art what is difficult to say with words. We compare our experiences with colleagues and investigate related fields to broaden our horizon. We use both standardised art-based assessments [1, 2] such as the Diagnostic Drawing Series [3], and less formal ones, according to the goals of the inquiry, the specific health care system we work with and our personal inclination [4]. There is also a vast area of projects dedicated to art-based research, in which knowledge is attained through artistic means and perceptual evidence [5, 6] while looking for new methods of investigation in resonance with the creative process [7].

In the field of "people prone to psychotic states" [8], evidence-based guidelines for clinical practice using art therapy have been compiled from quantitative and qualitative research, from academic literature, knowledge of experts as well as from art therapists' and users' experience and feedback. Their scope is to inform clinical work but also to help professionals develop further subjects for research projects. They comprise of 70 recommendations and they "make implicit processes explicit" ([4], p. 46), collecting information and building knowledge that covers three fundamental objectives for researchers: "making visible, making sense, making theory" ([5], p. 237).

As stated in the guidelines, art therapy is a non-threatening means of entering and maintaining a relationship. Participation in art therapy groups strengthens interpersonal relationships and contributes to the well-being of users [9, 10]. A research study about the beneficial results of group art therapy, conducted during the recent pandemic episode (March 2020) with the scope of measuring three items, motivation, participation, and social relationships, shows that users affected by psychotic states and by anxiety disorders benefit in terms of motivation and improve participation, while users affected by personality disorders and obsessive-compulsive

M. D. Cagnoletta (✉)
Art Therapy Italiana, Bologna, Italy

U. Volpe (ed.), *Arts Therapies in Psychiatric Rehabilitation*,
https://doi.org/10.1007/978-3-030-76208-7_2

disorders benefit in all areas (Moretti, A., in print). These kinds of assessments are done by taking into account the specific situation of the users, their context and not "on an interpretation of isolated images" ([7], p. 119).

Graphic expressions have been used as diagnostic tools for decades, but the outcome of these studies have no objective evidence [11]. However, Merlini ("Signs of Ill-being", unpublished findings) in a survey of 50 users hospitalised and referred for art therapy, observed how graphic elements and specific use of art materials may help to predict a profound and often sudden crisis leading to regressive behaviour and aggressive acting out. Before manifesting behavioural or mood changes, users on the verge of a psychotic breakdown change their style of painting and drawing. Art works can be the first witness of embodied suffering as well as "eloquent testimony" [12] of its healing capacity.

The first randomised controlled trial of group art psychotherapy with people diagnosed as schizophrenic [13], demonstrated a reduction of negative symptoms after only 12 weekly sessions. The model used for the trial followed the principles of group interactive art therapy [14] but it has been proved that another form of art therapy setting, the open art studio, provides benefits for users ([15], in print): the tangible aspect of making art, protecting and storing art works helps mediate the closeness and distance of social interactions while lessening catastrophic anxieties [16]. Art making conveys a sense of agency, while art therapy groups provide a safe place, where feelings of continuity and reliability are restored. The art therapy setting can became a healing place, while the use of rituals such as the circle of chairs at the end of the group or a group poem (Lombardi, personal communication) facilitate the passage from concrete thoughts to symbolisation. Art making is a source of both comfort and strength, as we can read in the work of outsider artists [17].

Due to the specific nature of our discipline, art works remain the primary element of enquiry that informs art therapy research. In order to enlarge our findings and promote vaster research projects, research methods must be inclusive and interdisciplinary, so that "the same creative skills art therapists use in practice can be applied to the design and conduct of research to contribute unique knowledge about the process, product, and outcomes of art therapy" ([5], p. 5).

References

1. Betts DJ. Art therapy assessment and rating instruments. Do they measure up? Arts Psychother. 2006;33(5):422–34.
2. Deaver SP. What constitutes art therapy research? Art Ther J Am Art Ther Assoc. 2002;19(1):23–7.
3. Cohen, Mills, Kijak. An introduction to the diagnostic drawing series. A standardised tool for diagnostic and clinical use. Art Ther J Am Art Ther Assoc. 1994;11(2):105–10.
4. Gilroy A. Art therapy, research and evidence-based practice. London: Sage Publications Ltd; 2006.
5. Kapitan L. Introduction to art therapy research. New York: Routledge; 2018.
6. Sullivan G. Art practice as research: inquiry in the visual arts. Thousand Oak, CA: Sage Publications; 2010.
7. McNiff S. Art-based research. London: Jessica Kingsley Publishers; 1998.

8. Brooker J, Cullum M, Gilroy A, McCombe B, Mahony J, Ringrose K, Russel D, Smart D, von Zeigbergk, Waldman J. The use of art work in art psychotherapy with people who are prone to psychotic states. An evidence-based clinical practice guideline. London: Goldsmiths, University of London; 2007.
9. Gilroy A, McNelly G. The changing shape of art therapy. London: Jessica Kingsley Publication; 2000.
10. Greenwood H, Layton G. Taking the piss, Inscape. Winter. 1991;7–14.
11. Burleigh L, Beutler L. A critical analysis of two creative arts therapies. Arts Psychother. 1997;23(5):375–81.
12. Adamson E. Art as healing. London: Conventure; 1990.
13. Richardson P, Jones K, Evans C, Stevens P, Rowe A. Exploratory RCT of art therapy as an adjunctive treatment in schizophrenia. J Mental Health. 2007;16(4):483–91.
14. Waller D. Group interactive art therapy. London: Routledge; 1993.
15. Masolini C, Bonamassa L, Chiovenda M, Fossi L. I gratificanti, esperienza di arteterapia nell'servizio psichiatrico di diagnosi e cura dell'ospedale di Prato. https://www.nuovarassegnastudipsichiatrici.it (in print, June 2021).
16. Killick, K. 1997, Unintegration and containment in acute psychosis. In Killick, K. & Schaverein, Psychotherapy and psychosis, Routledge, London.
17. Wojcik D. Outsider art. New York: Barnes and Nobles; 2016.

Commentary on the Conceptual Roots in Art Therapy: Rethinking Sublimation

3

Elizabeth Stone

Viganò and Magnotti's chapter reviewed the scope of visual art therapy from its sources in the late nineteenth century to the present day by including diverse theoretical approaches and practices in Europe, North America, and beyond. An admirably vast undertaking for a single chapter, the authors traced the fascinating historical antecedents of art therapy to its wide implementation today. Then, they introduced the reader to research initiatives, evaluating the efficacy of some models. They raised the question: what works in art therapy, for whom, and how? Addressing these questions across mental health population lines is valuable and calls upon us to consider how the art therapist is trained optimally to do the appropriate psychological or rehabilitative work required for his or her clinical population.

To comprehend such dense historical paths with only a few concise sentences for each, one can resonate fully only for those readers already versed in the history of art therapy and its contemporary offshoots. Further explanation for the newer reader necessitates filling in these gaps. My task in this commentary is to provide an alternative or complementary approach with an eye to the future direction of the field. In doing so, I hope to address one historical gap by offering an updating of my own.

Whether we divide the lens through which we view art therapy practice into the psychotherapeutic vs. the rehabilitative, as evinced by the authors, or advocate for an amalgam of the two, as in my own approach, much of our choice depends upon the comprehensiveness and depth of our training. It is our training and supervision that gives us the tools to think through new clinical needs and dilemmas, and figure out how to address them. This is different than simply amassing a set of therapeutic

E. Stone (✉)
Private Practice in Art Therapy and Psychoanalysis, Grenoble, France

Graduate Department of Art Therapy, New York University, New York, NY, USA

Ecole des Psychologues Praticiens, Lyon, France

Lyceum Academy, Milan, Italy

U. Volpe (ed.), *Arts Therapies in Psychiatric Rehabilitation*,
https://doi.org/10.1007/978-3-030-76208-7_3

techniques. Technique arises out of a relational comprehension based upon sound theory.

In my own evolution over the past 40 or so years, I recall vividly thinking as a beginner that if I only knew enough precise techniques with which to treat any given clinical problem, I would be a well-prepared art therapist. However, quite the opposite developed. Rather than to assert or impose my theoretical ideas, I have maintained readiness to be surprised by how the art therapeutic process unfolded. This changed the way I saw the therapeutic presence of my role: from myself as "knower" to that of "learner." Both my patients and I play necessarily different roles within the context of our co-created art therapy sessions.

After having identified my art therapy roots in ego psychology with my earliest mentor, Edith Kramer, as my knowledge of psychoanalytic literature broadened, I discovered some of its fascinating advances. Finding new compatibility with a developmental object relations approach, and then a self-psychology approach, in time new psychoanalytic evolution gave birth to the "relational movement" [1], which extended our thinking about the therapeutic relationship. We can now view it as arising within the interactive context, a co-created model akin to the early mother–infant interaction. As attachment theory gained ground, an interweaving of these ideas with art therapy principles became natural, congruent, and plausible.

We've heard the saying "everything old is new again." And so, I return to an old concept, "sublimation" in art therapy, to find new meaning [2]. Originally introduced by Kramer to describe how raw emotion and unbridled energy were transformed by the drives into culturally acceptable art expression [3], her explanation championed sublimation as the principal mechanism affirming art therapy as a valid therapeutic discipline. This earned the respect of the psychoanalytic community in the mid-twentieth century and provided the theoretical underpinnings of art therapy as distinguished from art teaching.

Since then, not only have many psychoanalysts questioned the veracity of sublimation itself, other practitioners had already debunked all psychoanalytic ideas, so dismissing sublimation was easy for them. Yet many people continued to express wonderment and awe at how the transformation of emotion, psychic trauma, and much more could become powerful expression and vibrant imagery. Via creativity, play, sometimes skill, and imagination, what is the mechanism underlying this transformation? And, how can we explain it intrapsychically in art therapy? Especially striking is that we continue to witness imagery brought forth by individuals in psychic disarray.

Although many considered sublimation if not outdated, fundamentally flawed or having outlived its usefulness, it has remained impossible to dismiss. Due to advances in psychoanalytic thinking, the drives no longer hold the same place of theoretical importance that they held in the first half of the twentieth century [4]. This has freed the concept of sublimation to embody transformational elements from other motivational systems. Rather than being only a product of conflict between the drives (libidinal and aggressive), sublimation can also be seen as arising out of affect, trauma, relational conflict, and the like.

Instead of viewing the art therapist as merely a benign witness to the sublimation process, we realize that the art product is created interactively. Beebe and Lachmann have reminded us "…inner experience is organized in the interactive context" ([5], p. 490). We understand the co-created mother–infant relationship as the prototype for the therapeutic relationship [6]. Even if the art therapist is silent, her presence as generator of the therapeutic action makes her a partner in fostering self-regulation, and hence, that which we can still call "sublimation."

References

1. Beebe B, Lachmann FM. The relational turn in psychoanalysis: a dyadic systems view from infant research. Contemp Psychoanal. 2003;39:379–409.
2. Stone E. Addendum – sublimation. In: Rubin JA, editor. Approaches to art therapy: theory and technique. 3rd ed. New York, NY: Routledge; 2016. p. 101–2.
3. Kramer E. Sublimation and art therapy. In: Rubin JA, editor. Approaches to art therapy: theory and technique. 2nd ed. New York, NY: Routledge; 2001. p. 28–39.
4. Freud S. The ego and the Id. The standard edition of the complete psychological works of Sigmund Freud (1914–1916). In: On the history of the psycho-analytic movement, papers on metapsychology and other works, vol. XIX. London, UK: Hogarth Press; 1923. p. 237–58.
5. Beebe B, Lachmann F. Co-constructing inner and relational processes: Self and mutual regulation in infant research and adult treatment. Psychoanal Psychol. 1998;15(4):480–516.
6. Beebe B, Lachmann FM. The contribution of mother–infant mutual influence to the origins of self- and object representation. Psychoanal Psychol. 1988;5:305–37.

4 Art Therapy in Mental Health Recovery: Towards an Expanded Lens

Patricia Fenner

Applications of art therapy in mental health commonly address treatment goals including symptom relief, management and reduction, psychosocial functioning and rehabilitation. A scoping review [1] identified health promotion and illness prevention as overarching domains of evidence-based art therapy. Research reviewed in this chapter reflects studies undertaken in Global North countries with sophisticated mental health systems able to provide nuanced levels of care. Increasingly in the USA, Australia, and the United Kingdom, adoption of the recovery values of connectedness, hope, identity, meaning in life, and empowerment has brought a strengths-based orientation to mental health [2].

One critical review identified benefits including self-discovery and expression, and improved social identity [3]. Evidence provided by people with lived experience of mental illness illuminates art making as transformative, supportive of taking control of one's life, and leading to increased self-confidence and determination [4] and as such relies less on specific diagnostic groupings, the approach preferred by Vigano and Magnotti. At this clinical level, a recent systematic review in the treatment of depression and anxiety [5] found moderate evidence for art associated with psychological trauma and limited evidence associated with physical trauma. Art therapy was found to be a positive adjunct to standard treatment in a study of 78 adults experiencing severe eating disorders who participated in a museum visiting program [6]. Results showed high levels of acceptability of art as a means of self-expression and creativity, though with no significant impacts on body image or preoccupations with eating. Processing intrusive memories and improving cognition are two goals of art therapy interventions amongst Veterans experiencing PTSD [7].

In recent years, the arts and health have gained ground in the Asia Pacific including addressing stigma [8] and trauma care following natural disaster [9]. The arts,

P. Fenner (✉)
School of Psychology and Public Health, La Trobe University, Melbourne, VIC, Australia
e-mail: P.Fenner@latrobe.edu.au

U. Volpe (ed.), *Arts Therapies in Psychiatric Rehabilitation*,
https://doi.org/10.1007/978-3-030-76208-7_4

and ill/health in Asia are understood in keeping with the roles they have played traditionally, notwithstanding broadscale influences of the "West" [10].

Specifically, art therapy in the service of mental health recovery has been adopted by some island states in the Pacific. Small scale qualitative studies indicate outcomes not dissimilar to other recovery settings, albeit with distinctive local qualities. A study of young adults experiencing mental illness participated in a year-long community-based art therapy program in Apai, Samoa. Here art was found to enhance a sense of identity and belonging, improve self-awareness, and reinforce a sense of self-value [11]. Early results from a similar cohort in Suva, Fiji revealed approval for art making across all stakeholder groups of mental health professionals, young adults with mental illness, and carers after engagement in therapeutic art making which emphasized traditional art materials [12].

In Terengganu, Malaysia a group art therapy program with women marginalized due to their divorced single parent status, found art provided an opportunity to explore and express feelings of loneliness, loss, and grief [13]. The release of long-held emotions led to enhanced self-awareness, improved self-esteem, and inner strength.

The findings from Asian studies are small scale and preliminary. Yet a significant function is performed in alerting us to an expanded global perspective in order to better understand the relevance, applicability, and value of art therapy in mental health rehabilitation and recovery.

References

1. Fancourt D, Finn S. What is the evidence on the role of arts in improving health and well-being? A scoping review. In: Health evidence network HEN synthesis report 67. Copenhagen: WHO Regional Office for Europe; 2019.
2. Stickley T, Wright N, Slade M. The art of recovery: outcomes from participatory art activities for people using mental health services. J Ment Health. 2018;27(4):367–73.
3. Van Lith T, Schofield MJ, Fenner P. Identifying the evidence base for arts-based practices and their potential benefit for mental health recovery: a critical review. Disabil Rehabil. 2013;35(16):1309–23. https://doi.org/10.3109/09638288.2012.732188.
4. Van Lith T, Fenner P, Schofield MJ. The lived experience of art making as a companion to the mental health recovery process. Disabil Rehabil. 2011;33(8):652–60.
5. McMillan J, Moo A, Arora R, Costa B. The clinical effectiveness and current practice of art therapy for trauma, evidence review. Melbourne: Worksafe, TAC, Monash University; 2018.
6. Thaler L, Drapeau C, Leclerc J, Lajeunesse M, Cottier D, Kahan E, Ferenczy N. An adjunctive, museum-based art therapy experience in the treatment of women with severe eating disorders. Arts Psychother. 2017;56:1–6.
7. Campbell M, Decker K, Kruk K, Deaver S. Art therapy and cognitive processing therapy for combated-related PTSD: a randomised controlled trial. Art Ther J Am Art Ther Assoc. 2016;33(1):160–77.
8. Potash JS, Ho RTH, Chick JKY, Au Yeung FSW. Viewing and engaging in an art therapy exhibit by people living with mental illness: implications for empathy and social change. Public Health. 2013;127(8):735–44.
9. Ho RTH, Fan F, Lai AHY, Lo PHY, Potash JS, Kalmanowitz DL, Nan JKM, Pon AKL, Shi Z, Chan CLW. An expressive arts-based and strength-focused experiential training

program for enhancing the efficacy of teachers affected by earthquake in China. Creat Educ. 2012;3(1):67–74. https://doi.org/10.4236/ce.2012.31011.
10. Kalmanowitz D, Potash JS, Chan SM, editors. Art therapy in Asia: to the bone or wrapped in silk. London and Philadelphia: Jessica Kingsley; 2012.
11. Fenner P, Ryan B, Latai L, Percival S. Art making and the promotion of wellbeing in Samoa—participants' lived experience of a recovery oriented intervention. Arts Health. 2018;10(2):124–37.
12. Ryan B, Fenner P, Chang O, Qaloewai S, Nabukavou T, Chetty S. Art making in mental health – a Fijian pilot study. Australas Psychiatry. 2021;29(2)
13. Fenner P, Mohamad Z. "What we have shared is actually a big secret": group art therapy with divorced single mothers in Malaysia. Art Ther J Am Art Ther Assoc. 2019;36:59–67.

Part II

Music Therapy

Music Therapy in Psychiatry

5

Emma Millard and Catherine Carr

5.1 Introduction

Music therapy has a long tradition of work in mental health care [1]. The World Federation of Music Therapy defines it as '… the professional use of music and its elements as an intervention in medical, educational, and everyday environments with individuals, groups, families, or communities who seek to optimize their quality of life and improve their physical, social, communicative, emotional, intellectual, and spiritual health and wellbeing. Research, practice, education, and clinical training in music therapy are based on professional standards according to cultural, social, and political contexts' [2].

5.2 History

The idea of music as being able to 'soothe the soul' is documented in ancient biblical and Greek texts, yet the contemporary music therapy profession was only recently formed in the last 50–70 years [3, 4]. The table below outlines historic examples of the use of music to heal the body and mind (Table 5.1):

The Second World War was a pivotal point for the music therapy profession: The importance of music as a therapeutic activity in the care of soldiers returning with 'shell-shock' (now recognised as post-traumatic stress disorder) led to a recognition of the value of music more generally in mental health care. Within the United

E. Millard (✉) · C. Carr
Unit for Social and Community Psychiatry, WHO Collaborating Centre for Mental Health Service Development, Queen Mary University of London, London, UK

Mental Health Care of Older Adults, East London NHS Foundation Trust, London, UK
e-mail: e.h.millard@qmul.ac.uk; c.e.carr@qmul.ac.uk

U. Volpe (ed.), *Arts Therapies in Psychiatric Rehabilitation*,
https://doi.org/10.1007/978-3-030-76208-7_5

Table 5.1 Historic examples of the uses of music to heal body and mind as cited by Odell-Miller [3] and McCaffrey [4]

~24,000 years BC	Music and healing depicted in cave paintings. Use by shamans	Suggests early recognition of therapeutic potential of music
~1000 years BC	Bible account of Saul being soothed by David playing the harp	Recognition of potential for music to calm and soothe emotional distress
~550 years BC	Pythagoras links musical notes to mathematical equations, leading to a theory of potential effects of music on the soul and impact of emotions of the listener	First clear use of music for therapeutic purposes
~350 years BC	Use of music in medicine to treat patients in 'Asclepion' healing temples	Music used as part of a holistic treatment for both psychological and physical ailments
~Fourth century	St Cecelia, patron saint of music	Recognition of the connection between music and emotions
~Fifth to fifteenth century middle ages	Therapeutic value of music recognised by Arabs and healing properties of music referred to in literature	
Fifteenth–eighteenth century	Article 'music physically considered' published Use of music to treat tarantism (thought to be caused by being bitten by a tarantula spider, resulting in delirium and an uncontrollable urge to dance). Composition of 'tarantellas' to accompany dancing and encourage fatigue to enable the person to then rest	One of the earliest accounts of the therapeutic use of music to specifically alleviate mental distress Early example of the properties of music (melodic line, repetition, increasing tempo) being used to impact upon a physical condition
Nineteenth century	Music groups and performances in hospitals and asylums. Use of phonograph to play music as a form of diversion. Illenau hospital in Germany: Use of music as an aesthetic and environmental means of bringing harmony to body and soul (Gemüth). Guild of St Cecilia formed in London, UK 1891—musicians performing in hospitals to aid healing. Strict protocols for performances including playing behind a screen	Recognition of potential of music to distract; valuing of the aesthetic; provide occupational therapy; socialisation opportunities afforded by making music in groups. Introduction of governance and control in the use of music in medical settings

Kingdom (UK), formation of the National Health Service in 1948 created a climate in which services could be designed anew, with a focus on free and accessible healthcare for all. Within this context, the overcrowded and institutionalised environments of asylums were challenged and over the following 40 years, a move was made to integrate mental health and general hospital provision, with a focus on providing care within the community [5, 6]. At this same point in time, the randomised controlled trial became the new 'gold standard' in providing evidence for medical interventions [7].

The emergence of the contemporary music therapy profession was within this new context of hope and possibility. The first UK training course in music therapy was established by Juliette Alvin in 1968 with both herself and an early student, Mary Priestley, documenting their work in psychiatric hospitals [8–10]. McCaffrey [4] notes that as the medical profession began to take interest in music therapy, this was viewed with scepticism and suspicion by some and may have resulted in a drive to provide systematic and experimental evidence for its effects. Whilst for some, the value of music was unequivocal, the pressures on services (particularly within the 1980s–1990s) led to posts being frozen or cut [3] and an urgent need across arts therapies professions to provide research evidence that underpinned their work.

More recent developments in music therapy have been influenced by wider political movements in mental health (for example, service user involvement and the recovery model), technological advances enabling recording and use of computer software [11, 12] and collaboration and interdisciplinary work with wider arts therapists, psychologists and multi-disciplinary teams [13–17].

5.3 Basic Principles and Techniques

As with all of the arts therapies, music therapy practice is underpinned by theories from both wider psychotherapy and those more specific to the art-form itself, many of which were incorporated and developed in the 1950s as music therapists sought to describe and develop their work. Whilst the World Federation for Music Therapy suggests five main models (Benenzon, Bonny method of Guided Imagery in Music, Behavioural, Nordoff-Robbins and Analytical Music Therapy), others have suggested up to 11 (including Community, Resource-Oriented, Culture-centred, Aesthetic, Vocal psychotherapy, feminist, psychodynamic, developmental and anthroposophical music therapy) [18]. At its heart, much practice is underpinned by humanistic and person-centred with principles of enabling client potential, and aspects of empathy, congruence and unconditional positive regard of key importance [19]. As music therapists became embedded within psychiatric hospitals, many saw the value in emerging ideas from psychoanalytic and psychodynamic schools which provided a language and framework to understand the relationships and nonverbal interactions as they develop and evolve through musical interplay [3, 20]. Of particular importance are Bion's writing on containment—which in musical terms can include providing a musical structure to support increased arousal, reduce anxiety and offer form to chaotic or fragmented play; and Winnicott's writing of the importance of play, creativity and potential space [21]. Within the United States, the predominance of behavioural models has influenced the way in which music therapy is applied to meet specific goals, within the framework of behavioural motivation, achievement, psychoeducation and reward [22, 23]. In contrast, music therapists trained in Paul Nordoff and Clive Robbins' methods [24] have applied a music-centred understanding to their work whereby improvised and active music-making is seen as the core agent of therapeutic action and change [3, 25].

Music therapy continues to develop theoretical models and practice in line with current contexts. More recent developments are influenced by 'third wave' approaches including mentalisation [26], cognitive analytic [27, 28] and mindfulness [29]. Concurrently, there is an increased emphasis upon the role of relationships and attachment. Trondalen has developed a theory of relational music therapy, influenced by the work of Daniel Stern and Colwyn Trevarthen [30, 31]. She outlines how understanding the role of nonverbal interactions between mother and baby in early life can help to underpin the ways in which music therapy can support formation of identity and relationships in both active and receptive contexts.

Of particular importance to music therapy in psychiatry in the last couple of decades, is the turn towards resource and recovery oriented frameworks. Rolvsjord highlights the importance of acknowledging and working with client strengths and abilities in mental health care and underscores the relevance of rebalancing the therapeutic relationship to ensure this is equal, collaborative and mutually trusting [32]. Her work forms the foundation of more recent music therapy practice within a recovery framework [33] which underscores the importance of valuing client's own expertise and knowledge about their health, and emphasises the value of connectedness, hope, identity, meaning and empowerment (CHIME) in living with and recovering a life from mental illness [34].

Despite the range of techniques and models within music therapy, all share a commonality in the sense that music, and the relationships developed within this, are the basis for change. The contextual model of psychotherapy [35] suggests that client and therapist belief in the therapy, client motivation to change and the therapeutic relationship developed are more important for change than the specific therapeutic model alone. This model suggests that music therapy may be right for some, but not all clients. An understanding of factors that facilitate or hinder engagement may help us to better understand 'for whom' music therapy may best be for and 'when'.

Theories regarding the development of self are pivotal across all models of music therapy—both active/expressive and receptive [30]. The impact of early interactional relationships upon our development of understanding of self and others naturally helps to underscore the relational benefits afforded by music therapy. The ways in which caregivers and infants coordinate and interact nonverbally demonstrate ways in which music can aid self-regulation, awareness of feeling states and development of theory of mind [36, 37].

Importantly, Trondalen [30] underscores core, shared principles of music therapy practice (Table 5.2):

Such processes can clearly be linked to many issues faced by clients living with mental illness across different stages and life courses. Here, arousal and regulation, managing and naming different emotions, building relationships, creating new narratives and identities and identifying ways music can be a health resource are of prime importance. Such shared features suggest that there are processes that cut across diagnostic subgroups and are shared by mental health service users as a

Table 5.2 Core principles of music therapy (MT) practice

MT is interactional and interactive—never a 'doing to'	MT utilises creativity as a means of adapting to and overcoming challenges
MT harnesses neurological and physiological effects of music: brain and timing/movement/motivation; mood and arousal/stress regulation; bonding and feeling together	MT enables formation and development of relationships via primarily nonverbal means in new contexts (which in a community setting promotes development of social capital); [38–40]
MT promotes engagement and recovery	

whole [41]. In contrast, there is evidence for specific features of musical interaction in psychosis [42, 43], suggesting that diagnostic-specific processes may also play a role. The extent to which music therapists focus upon diagnostic specificity versus wider shared features has yet to be determined. Understanding of both may help to disentangle when individual or diagnostic-specific groups may be more appropriate, or not across different care pathways.

There is good evidence that music therapy can engage and motivate clients [44, 45] which may link to the neurological processes of reward associated in listening to and participating in music [46]. The nonverbal interactions through active improvisatory music-making provide a means of relating and regulating interactions when words fail [30]. Evolutionary psychology suggests music evolved as a social practice and there is evidence that music-making promotes bonding and relationships with others [47, 48], particularly through singing [49]. This in turn can support wider social and community connection [39, 40, 50, 51]. The creativity involved in producing or responding to music enables a means of trying new ideas, taking risks, play [21] and experiencing different ways of knowing—both implicit and explicit [30]. Properties of music, such as timing, tempo and harmonic progression can be used sensitively to help clients regulate their interactions with others [52]. This is important when considering the challenge of doing so for example, either through a manic or psychotic episode. We know that when making music, much wider and more diverse neurological processes are used compared to speaking alone [46]. There is thus the opportunity to integrate physical and emotional processes; cognition need not be the primary mode of relating [30]. Finally, music therapy can provide a different, strengths-based experience which, in community settings, has potential to reduce stigma and more broadly, can be culturally appropriated [50, 51]. Such resource-oriented ways of working [32, 53] are in line with wider concepts of recovery in mental health, and value the process of recovering one's own identity, hope and connection to others [33].

Music therapy is provided within individual and group formats. The format is influenced by setting, service and point within the care pathway and often adapted to meet specific needs within this. For example, within an acute ward environment, traditional therapeutic boundaries are 'looser' in the sense that group members may be allowed to come and go during a session, but the level of activity, direction and structure from the therapist is greater to provide a sense of safety and means of supporting engagement [54]. This differs to individual work in a community setting, where boundaries may be reinforced and thought about to a greater degree, and where there may be greater flexibility and freedom in the way music is used.

The main techniques in music therapy can be thought about as either active/expressive (actively making and producing music together through improvisation, playing known songs or songwriting/composition) or receptive (listening to music either live or recorded).

5.3.1 Music Listening and Receptive Methods

At its most simple, music listening may be used to build a sense of safety and rapport early on in therapy with music appreciation and discussion groups having a particular value on acute inpatient wards. However, more formalised and structured approaches also exist, influenced by the extensive clinical practice and research of Helen Bonny [55], who developed the practice of Guided Imagery in Music. This method involves a relaxation induction to facilitate an altered state of consciousness and then listening to a programme of music, selected by the therapist. The client dialogues with the therapist whilst listening, sharing any images, experiences or sensations evoked by the music. Afterwards, time is taken to return to waking consciousness, reflect upon the imagery and integrate this with wider life. Mandala drawing may be used to facilitate this transition. Whilst the full form of the Bonny Method of Guided Imagery in Music (BMGIM) is contraindicated for some psychiatric diagnoses (for example, acute psychosis), there have been many adaptations to address and support specific needs of psychiatric populations [56–61]. In an observational study, Wrangsjö and Körlin reported favourable symptom-based and interpersonal outcomes of BMGIM in community outpatients [62]. Körlin has also developed a method of 'music breathing' to support clients with complex PTSD [63].

Psychoeducational approaches attempt to increase the knowledge and improve illness-management for psychiatric patients. They have been implemented in single-session models and incorporate cognitive-behavioural principles [64]. Lyric analysis gives an opportunity for patients to reflect on their own experiences and relationships [22]. Songwriting techniques have been used to increase hope and motivation [65], or to work with families post-discharge [23] and music listening programmes have been used to reduce stress and anxiety in older adults [66].

One new method being developed is the use of personalised playlists for people with dementia. It is hoped that this approach could help to tackle agitation and medication adherence and help older people to live independently in their own home for longer [67].

5.3.2 Musical Improvisation and Active Methods

Clinical improvisation is where the client(s) and therapist create music together, in the moment. Unlike other types of musical improvisation, the therapist uses their role in the music to support, enhance and encourage musical development and uses specific musical techniques to support, highlight, expand upon, provide structure or contain [68]. The improvisation may be structured to focus upon different roles (e.g. one person leads the improvisation in a group), thematic (e.g. to explore an emotion or situation) or free (no instructions given and created in the moment). The music created is viewed as a communication of the relationship developing between client(s) and therapist and in many models, is discussed afterwards as a means of reflecting upon and integrating the experience, emotions and relations that evolved.

Music already known to clients has value in building rapport between individuals and can be a means of sharing an aspect of one's identity or feeling state. Sharing of known songs is of particular importance in work with dementia clients where the musical memory allows engagement in the moment, with others and a sense of achievement and connection [69, 70].

Songwriting has been used to support clients in processing their life experiences, both individually and in groups [71–73]. Music therapists often work collaboratively with clients, taking joint responsibility for the creation of both the lyrics and the music in the songwriting process [74]. Songwriting may provide a way for clients to access inner feeling and put those feelings into words [45, 75]. A song structure can offer containment for difficult experiences, meaning that patients are able to share more within the context of the therapeutic relationship, e.g. using the 12-bar blues [76, 77]. Both songwriting and composition provide a means of recording an aspect of the therapy and can be an important source of recognition and achievement for clients, as well as a means of communicating about mental illness to the wider world [78].

A survey of 23 European music therapists found that supportive psychotherapy and psychoanalytically informed approaches to music therapy were most frequently used in psychiatry, whilst techniques of free improvisation with minimal or talking/verbal interpretation were used most frequently across all diagnoses. Composed songs were used more frequently with schizophrenia and bipolar disorders whilst techniques utilising symbolic thinking (such as musical role play or play rules) were more frequent for non-psychotic disorders [79].

5.4 Available Evidence

5.4.1 Schizophrenia and Psychosis

It has been suggested that music therapy can help people with schizophrenia through making sense of a chaotic internal world. The transition from repetitive, sensorial play to the use of musical form has been seen as an important goal of music therapy with this client group [42]. A recent Cochrane review looking at music therapy for people with schizophrenia and schizophrenia-like illnesses concluded that there seem to be benefits for patients' global state, mental state, functioning and quality of life over a short to medium term [80]. Eighteen trials were included in this review with a total of 1215 participants and the evidence was found to be of low to moderate quality. Group therapy was used in most of the included studies and almost all were conducted in inpatient settings. One major concern was that a number of studies offered music therapy interventions which were implemented by staff with minimal music therapy training, e.g. nurses or psychiatrists.

A non-experimental follow-up study in Germany found that patients were able to engage in rhythmical attunement during initial sessions, which was associated with a decrease in psychotic symptoms [81]. This study has a number of limitations, primarily that there was no control group with which to compare results. It also had a small sample size (n = 21) and offered a relatively small number of sessions (n = 5). Another study used a specific approach—Music Therapy incorporated into Cognitive Remediation (MTCR) for patients in the community who attended a 30-session programme. They found significant decrease in symptoms, although there was no control group to compare with and the assessors were not blinded to the aims of the project [82].

As well as the randomised controlled trials (RCTs) included in the Cochrane review, a small number of qualitative studies have looked at the experiences of patients with schizophrenia who have attended music therapy. In a meta-synthesis, Solli and Rolvsjord [83] found four superordinate themes which were integral to patients' experiences: freedom, contact, well-being and symptom relief; patients reported finding the sessions enjoyable, engaging and motivating, which is a promising finding for people who may be experiencing negative symptoms such as apathy and emotional flatness. A case study from the same author documents the improvements he saw in a single patient with psychosis: the patient attended 28 sessions in an inpatient setting and the therapist observed a number of positive changes which generalised to outside the therapy setting [84]. A further study of pivotal moments in music therapy, supplemented by a case study, suggested that in adult mental health, such moments are characterised by alteration of time perception, capacity to deal with 'here and now' and emotional expression of the experience [85].

A modified form of Guided Imagery and Music (GIM) has been trialled with a small number of patients with psychosis (n = 9) in Denmark. The patients attended a slow open group over the course of around 6 months. The therapists adapted the sessions to be more structured for this client group and used shorter music programmes. The patients reported the group to be supportive and appreciated the structured format. Eight out of the nine patients reported feeling satisfied with the treatment [86].

The results from trials and qualitative studies suggest a promising trend of music therapy being helpful for patients with schizophrenia. Larger, higher quality studies will be essential in the future, as well as further investigation of patient experiences of music therapy.

5.4.2 Depression and Anxiety

It has been suggested that people with depression are likely to engage with music therapy because music-making provides a social, pleasurable and meaningful activity [87]. A Cochrane review examining music therapy for depression concluded that music therapy provides short-term benefits for depression symptoms in comparison to treatment as usual. Engagement in music therapy is also associated with decreased anxiety levels and improved functioning for those with depression [88]. Nine studies were included in the review with a total of 421 participants. Five studies were conducted in mental health services, two were with older adults in care homes and two were in high schools. Three studies evaluated anxiety symptoms in the short term as well as depression symptoms.

A systematic review was conducted by Zhao and colleagues to look at the effects of music therapy for older adults with depression [89]. They used broader inclusion criteria for what constitutes music therapy than the Cochrane review and found 19 studies to include in the review. They found evidence that music therapy plus standard therapies favoured standard therapies alone. However, they did not find an effect of music therapy when compared to standard therapies alone.

CBT-Music was explored in a feasibility trial in Canada with 28 participants. They found that recruitment, retention and acceptability were high, but there were minimal effects of the intervention on anxiety and depression symptoms [90]. The intervention was based on a group CBT guided self-help structure. Music was incorporated through known songs as themes, re-writing popular song lyrics to reflect experiences of anxiety and depression, lyric analysis, thought records (about songs) and behavioural experiments (such as playing an instrument). The groups were facilitated by mental health crisis workers with a musical background.

Studies often combine depression and anxiety treatment as these are seen as common mental health conditions. There is limited literature looking at music therapy for anxiety alone. A study in the USA found that clinical improvisation was effective in the treatment of anxiety for 16 participants. Their anxiety symptoms were compared from baseline to week 6 and to week 12 of treatment. A significant reduction in anxiety symptoms over time was found [91]. Another study found that receptive and active methods of music therapy were effective in reducing anxiety and depression levels for patients with generalised anxiety disorder [92]. This study had a very small sample size of only seven participants. Bidabadi and colleagues looked at music therapy for patients with obsessive compulsive disorder (OCD) in Iran. Thirty participants demonstrated a larger decrease in obsessive symptoms, anxiety symptoms and depression symptoms when they received receptive music therapy 3 days per week as opposed to standard treatment alone [93].

One study has looked at the qualitative experiences of music therapy participants who were experiencing depression. It was found that patients experienced songwriting groups as a happy and safe place where they were able to explore difficult feelings through lyric generation. The participants reported an increased motivation to join creative groups in the community. It was also highlighted that the ending of the groups led to a sense of loss and hopelessness for some [75].

Finding meaning and pleasure could be an important factor in the 'effectiveness' of music therapy for patients who often report feelings of worthlessness and being without a sense of purpose. There is also the potential for music therapy to help manage symptoms of anxiety. Further high-quality research, including understanding of patient experiences, is essential for this field.

5.4.3 Dementia

Music therapy is often used in dementia settings to decrease the behavioural and psychological symptoms of dementia (BPSD). Recent meta-analyses have found a positive impact of music therapy interventions on agitation, anxiety and disruptive behaviours [89, 94]. When music therapy was offered for more than three months, a stronger effect on the reduction of anxiety levels was observed [95]. In the most recent, meta-analysis 34 trials were eligible, including RCTs, cohort designs and crossover trials. Music therapy was found to have a significant effect on disruptive behaviour and anxiety. Other outcomes included cognitive function, depression and quality of life, all of which trended towards improvement with music therapy treatment but were non-significant [89].

One study ($n = 55$) in Northern Italy found group music therapy to be effective in reducing BPSD when compared to education or activity groups. The improvements were maintained at the one-month follow-up point [96]. The same author then undertook a study looking at three one-month cycles of music therapy, with a month's gap in between. Sixty participants were enrolled and they found those in the music therapy group experienced significantly reduced delusions, agitation and apathy compared to the control group of standard care [97]. More recently, Raglio and colleagues conducted a larger study ($n = 120$) examining the effects of active music therapy or personalised music listening in comparison to treatment as usual. They found an improvement in BPSD in all three groups, with no significant advantage for the treatment groups [98]. The authors suggest that the high levels of dropout (18%) and a low number of sessions ($n = 20$) may have contributed to this finding. Thornley tested group music therapy against active engagement groups on an acute psychiatric dementia ward. They found no evidence that music therapy was more effective in reducing symptoms than the active engagement intervention. The authors cite their small sample size as a major limitation ($n = 16$) [99].

Individual music therapy has been found to decrease agitation and disruptiveness in patients with dementia and reduce the likelihood that they will need a higher dose of medication [100]. Participants were assigned to bi-weekly individual music therapy for 6 weeks, or treatment as usual. The authors suggest that carrying out the intervention in a short space of time meant that the natural degenerative effects of dementia were not so pronounced, so it was possible to detect improvements in agitation. It was also recommended that levels of prescribed medication are more commonly measured as an indicator of the effectiveness of psychosocial interventions for those with dementia. Another feasibility trial of individual music therapy for dementia attempted to involve carers through video presentations of the therapy. The authors concluded that the intervention was feasible and shows promise as an approach. Further research into individual, weekly active music-making sessions is recommended [101].

Outcome measures in dementia studies often rely on caregiver perspectives, who are unlikely to be blinded to the treatment condition. The Music in Dementia Assessment Scale (MiDAS) has been developed as a validated tool for observing the effects of music therapy. This checklist asks the rater to score patients in the following five areas: levels of interest, response, initiation, involvement and enjoyment. They are also asked if they noticed major changes in eight areas: vocal agitation, physical aggression, withdrawal, tearfulness, anxiety, laughter, enthusiasm and/or relaxed mood. A space for comments are also provided [102, 103]. A small study in Germany ($n = 9$) used time-series video evaluation to examine the effects of individual music therapy for patients with dementia. Compared to baseline scores, they found a significant improvement in communication behaviour, situational well-being and their expression of positive emotions [104].

At the time of writing this chapter, a large international RCT is underway. The Homeside study will be looking at the effectiveness of training carers to implement musical interventions to target BPSD. The study will recruit 495 pairs of participants from five countries across the world and the music intervention will be compared with standard care plus a reading intervention, and standard care alone [105].

There is strong evidence that music therapy is effective in reducing behavioural and psychological symptoms in patients who have dementia, and that this is maintained over time. There are some difficulties in conducting participatory research with this group of people due to their symptoms, and a reliance on caregivers' or therapists' opinions. However, arts-based methods could be well placed to overcome some of these challenges. Future trials will help us to further understand the mechanisms of change in music therapy for people with dementia.

5.4.4 Trauma, PTSD and Refugees

A study in Norway estimated that 91% of psychiatric patients admitted to an inpatient unit had experienced trauma [106]. Given the role of trauma in precipitating or maintaining mental illness, practitioners in psychiatric settings are likely to work with patients in a way that is trauma-informed [107].

Veterans and refugees are populations which are particularly affected by post-traumatic stress disorder (PTSD). It has been estimated that 9% of refugees who are settled in Western countries have a diagnosis of PTSD [108]. Estimates of PTSD prevalence in veterans vary from 2% to 17% [109]. A systematic review of creative arts therapies for PTSD found that the quality of evidence was low, with only two studies looking at the effects of music therapy for PTSD [110]. Only one RCT looking at active music-making with patients with PTSD has been conducted and the study found significant reduction of symptoms for those engaged in a manualised music therapy group versus those in a control group [111]. The other study used music listening with limited therapist contact and found no significant effect on PTSD symptoms [112]. A theoretical review suggested that music therapy may be well placed to address the symptoms of negative affect and mood alterations for patients with PTSD [113].

Case studies have recorded music therapists' experiences of working with people whose primary diagnosis is directly related to the trauma they have experienced. One author suggested that GIM assisted eight Vietnam veterans to explore their inner lives and reconnect with their emotions in a safe way [114]. In another case study the importance of silence and musical form was explored [115]. In interviews with traumatised soldiers, group drumming was found to create feelings of openness, togetherness, sharing, closeness, connectedness and intimacy. Although the loud sounds of the drums were sometimes associated with the frightening war sounds that the soldiers had experienced, the soldiers described 'drumming out the rage' and regaining a sense of control [116].

More recently, guided imagery methods have shown promise in treating PTSD symptoms for refugees. A pilot study with 16 adult refugees found pre–post measures of sleep quality, well-being and social function demonstrated significant changes with large effect sizes. Evaluation of the single sessions showed that participants found the therapy acceptable and helpful and the authors suggest a larger-scale trial in this area is warranted [117]. Maack also found significant improvements for women with complex PTSD when treated with 50 hours of outpatient trauma therapy with the Bonny method of GIM. Participants reported feeling that the music in GIM could be a teacher, a keeper of knowledge or abilities, could model different kinds of relationships, it could be a space for different experiences, represent dissociated parts, bring or evoke imagery and be a connection with beauty or non-violent parts of the world [118].

There is limited, but promising evidence for the use of music therapy specifically with people who have experienced trauma, despite it being such a common experience in the psychiatric population. This field would benefit from further investigation into receptive methods such as GIM, which have shown promise in reducing symptoms of PTSD.

5.4.5 Eating Disorders

Music therapy for people who have a diagnosis of an eating disorder has not been well researched. A number of mechanisms for how music therapy could help those with an eating disorder have been proposed, such as the client experiencing holding and containment of their feelings which they may have missed out on as a child. Compulsive behaviour can be addressed through the use of rhythm and expression of the true self through musical play [119]. Robarts and Sloboda noted their observations of patients with eating disorders, including a tendency to play rapidly, without phrases, and a noticeable lack of warmth or flexibility in the music-making [120].

One RCT has examined the effect of music therapy on post-meal anxiety for patients with anorexia nervosa. Eighteen patients attended two music therapy groups per week after lunch. Their post-meal anxiety was tested on days that they attended music therapy and days which they did not. It was found that their anxiety was significantly reduced on the days which they attended the music therapy group [121].

In two case studies of music therapy with women diagnosed with eating disorders, the authors suggest that music therapy helped the patients by promoting health through musical experiences, and the relational musical experience created a link between the body and the mind [122].

A study in the USA contacted 19 eating disorder units to find out more about their treatment programmes. All of them offered arts-based treatments at least once per week. The authors suggest that, given the prevalence of arts-based treatments for eating disorders, further research is imperative to understand how and why arts therapies may, or may not be helpful for this client group [123].

5.4.6 Personality Disorders

There are limited research studies which engage participants with personality disorders. This may, in part, be because of the idea that patients with personality disorders need a different approach in their treatment. Mentalisation has been put forward as a framework which could be helpful for addressing distress in patients with personality disorders [124] and has received some attention in music therapy practice [26, 125].

A very small-scale feasibility trial has recently been published. Four participants with personality disorders undertook 40 sessions of music therapy. Their attendance was mostly good and the participants demonstrated some positive change. It is recommended that a larger-scale trial in this area would be feasible [126].

Music therapy has been proposed as a safe place to explore aggression for those with personality disorders [127]. Strehlow and Lindner reviewed their clinical notes for work with 20 patients with personality disorders. They found 10 interactional patterns associated with music therapy for these patients [128]. The authors hope that their findings will be the springboard for further research into music therapy with people with personality disorders. In a case study of a forensic patient with personality disorder, Short refers to the interactional patterns as a useful tool for thinking about music therapy with this client group [129].

Patients with personality disorders are often excluded from trials due to the specific nature of their symptoms; however, as alternative methods are being explored clinically with this group, further research in this area is imperative.

5.4.7 Addiction and Substance Misuse

A systematic review examining the effects of music therapy and music based interventions on substance misuse found 34 quantitative and six qualitative studies. Most interventions were found to be delivered in a group format and 26 of them were classified as music therapy. Motivation, depression, enjoyment, withdrawal and craving and music therapy helpfulness, locus of control, participation and coping skills were examined. The summaries suggest there is evidence for the effectiveness of music therapy or music based interventions over the control groups. In the qualitative studies, four general themes were identified: music served as a tool for expression of thoughts and feelings, music interventions facilitated group cohesion and relationships, music interventions were useful for learning skills regarding music, problem solving and social interaction, and the music interventions were associated with improved well-being and quality of life [130].

Another recent systematic review sought to look at the effectiveness of arts therapies in treating substance misuse disorders. The review included all types of creative arts therapies in the inclusion criteria; however, the only suitable studies were five music therapy studies. A meta-analysis was not possible due to high heterogeneity in approaches and outcomes measured; however, the results indicated that music therapy has a positive effect on substance misuse symptoms [131].

Gardstrom et al. [132] looked at the impact of group music therapy on levels of negative affect for participants with substance use disorders and mental illness. Twenty sessions of music therapy were provided on an inpatient unit and 89 survey responses were collected (from 49 patients). The authors tested for improvement in sadness, anxiety and anger. One-third of the participants experienced an improvement in all three affective states. This study has a number of limitations including the use of a non-validated measure. The group therapists also collected the data, which could have led to biased responses from the participants.

Overall the evidence for music therapy with patients who have substance misuse disorders seems promising but would benefit from further larger-scale studies. Music therapy may be helpful for reducing substance misuse symptoms and other psychiatric symptoms, as well as improving other skills and quality of life.

5.4.8 Perinatal Mental Health

Perinatal psychiatry has started to gain more attention in the past few years. The perinatal period has been defined in a number of ways; the WHO states it commences at 22 completed weeks of gestation and ends seven completed days after birth [133]. The NHS states that the perinatal period continues for one year after the birth of a child and may affect up to 20% of women [134]. There are a number of ways in which music therapy could be helpful for women experiencing perinatal mental health difficulties [135] but very little research has been conducted in this field.

Music therapists in a perinatal unit in the USA implemented the use of lullabies to work with new mothers with mental illness and their babies. The authors wrote about how the sessions included understanding how parents were using music in their lives, brainstorming about lullabies patients knew, identifying signs of babies' distress or overstimulation, writing a lullaby, choosing soothing activities to do whilst singing lullabies, and choosing calming music for babies. This was not a research trial, but the authors report a positive experience and recommend further investigation in this area [136].

5.4.9 Forensic Psychiatry

A systematic review and meta-analysis found five studies about music therapy for offenders. It reported positive effects of music therapy on self-esteem and social functioning, and that effect on depression and anxiety was related to the number of sessions offered; more than 20 sessions of music therapy gave a significantly stronger effect than fewer than 20 sessions [137]. The authors urge the reader to interpret results with caution as there were such a small number of included studies and they were of variable quality. The included studies offered a range of number of sessions in a variety of formats, i.e. individual, group and both.

Case studies have demonstrated the ways in which music therapy may be helpful for forensic patients. Loth noted that a music therapy group with male offenders seemed to be a place where they could express a choice and start to explore their 'negative' behaviours in a safe space [138]. The use of rap composition and recording has been suggested as a helpful way for forensic patients to channel aggressive feelings and improve congruency between emotions and behaviours. This approach also seems to motivate an often unmotivated population [139]. Compton-Dickenson has developed a cognitive analytic music therapy approach with forensic patients with personality disorders. She suggests that cognitive analytic therapy and music therapy can be combined to help patients with emotional regulation and accessing unbearable feelings [28].

It seems as though music therapy could be helpful for addressing 'negative' behaviour as well as clinical symptoms for people with a forensic history. Research into this area is particularly challenging, given the highly regulated environments for work, adaptations required to practice safely and the much longer duration of time required. Further research might also consider ways in which music therapy integrates with other disciplines in these settings.

5.4.10 Child and Adolescent Mental Health

The last meta-analysis looking at music therapy for children and adolescents with mental health conditions was conducted in 2004. Eleven studies were included in the analysis and a significant medium to large effect of music therapy was found [140]. The studies included in this review were of variable quality; some were not randomised and the diagnoses and interventions were often not described in much detail. Some of the studies included clients with developmental disorders.

Empirical evidence for music therapy with children in a psychiatry setting is growing. It has been found that music therapy combined with CBT was superior to treatment as usual in reducing anxiety symptoms in 36 children aged 8–12 years old [141]. Music therapy groups have been found to significantly improve mood rating scores in an adolescent psychiatric hospital in an observational study. This study involved a large number of participants ($n = 352$) who undertook standardised measures of mood before and after participating in a music therapy group [142]. A large-scale trial in Northern Ireland ($n = 251$) found mixed results. Music therapy was not found to have additional benefits compared to a control group for social skills after 13 weeks of treatment. However, there was an effect when the children were aged 13 or over. Self-esteem and depression scores significantly improved for the treatment group but there was no difference in family or social functioning [143].

In a family psychiatric treatment programme, Oldfield and colleagues found that, although it was often the children's behaviour that led to a referral to music therapy, the relationship between the parents and children usually became the focus of the work. Nonverbal improvised music-making and playful exchanges were a key aspect of developing communication between the parents and children [144].

Rap music has been reported as being helpful for adolescents with mental health conditions. Rap music may provide a gateway to accessing therapy and lyric generation can be a method of processing traumatic life experiences [145].

A quality improvement project in Canada asked adolescents to rate their experiences of a music therapy group. The young people ($n = 72$) reported that music therapy groups were helpful for elevating their mood, reducing anxiety and helpful in communicating and interacting. A small number reported that they did not find the groups helpful, and others said they had felt nervous, shy or awkward [146].

5.4.11 Mixed-Diagnosis Groups

Music therapy has been examined with heterogeneous diagnostic groups, as this is the most common approach to clinical work in psychiatric services. For outpatients in the community, music therapy has been used to target proactive coping skills. There was no significant improvement for the group who accessed music therapy versus psychoeducational groups, although qualitative data implied that patients in both groups often used music as a coping skill [147].

There is also a place for music therapy in working with people who are homeless and experiencing mental illness. A case study documented the use of the voice with men who were using a homeless shelter and had mental health conditions. The author noted the importance of doing something creative, meaningful and productive with others, which met some of the men's emotional needs in the context of a genuine relationship [148].

In Australia, Grocke and colleagues conducted a trial looking at songwriting groups for community patients. The group who engaged with music therapy experienced a significant improvement in their quality of life and spirituality scores compared to the standard care group [45]. Songwriting has been studied by Silverman and Baker in inpatient units, who found a positive and significant correlation between the flow and meaningfulness in songwriting and therapeutic outcomes [149]. They have developed a Meaningfulness in Songwriting Scale (MSS) to examine this relationship further [150].

Music therapy has been trialled alongside medication and found to be associated with a reduced need for neuroleptics in psychiatric care [151]. This potential effect of music therapy treatment has not been investigated before although it could be an emerging area of interest.

Music therapy inpatient work with patients with mixed diagnoses has been studied extensively. A systematic review in 2013 identified 98 papers reporting on music therapy with psychiatric inpatients. Thirty five of those were research studies with the rest being case studies. Particular challenges were reported in working with such a high patient turnover. Approaches to music therapy were diverse, depending on training of therapists and country of the study. The authors concluded that, although there were some indications of positive effects of music therapy, the studies were often of poor quality with low sample sizes, meaning that definitive conclusions were limited [54].

Silverman has conducted a high number of small-scale studies looking at the effects of music therapy in psychiatric settings. He has found limited significant quantitative results, likely due to small sample sizes, but often reports a positive trend for those who engage in music therapy groups. His studies explored a number of different outcomes for family-based educational music therapy [23] and educational music therapy groups [22, 65, 152].

One study looked at the effects of single-session active music therapy, receptive music therapy and CBT on mood state. They found that participants in the receptive music therapy group demonstrated larger improvements in mood than in the other two groups, although all three groups showed some improvement [153]. Another study in the USA compared music therapy groups on an acute inpatient unit to treatment as usual. The groups occurred three times per week and a total of 32 patients were involved in the study. They found greater improvements in quality of life for patients who attended the music therapy group. Satisfaction and perceived helpfulness were high for both groups. The music therapy group was reported to be more volatile than other standard care groups, with increased conflict amongst members. However, the authors suggest that this may have been a therapeutically useful process [154].

Studies which examine music therapy for diagnostically heterogeneous groups are likely to better represent actual clinical practice across different psychiatric settings and thus indicate more pragmatic research designs. The setting of the work has an important bearing on how music therapy is provided: Community and inpatient work rely upon very different aims, approaches and processes. This underscores the importance of sensitivity to the local setting, culture and context. Future studies may seek to gain a better understanding of the shared features across different psychiatric diagnoses and how specific music therapy techniques might best support these within a group context.

5.4.12 Experiences of Inpatient Music Therapy

MacDonald [155] found 16 themes in interviews with psychiatric inpatients who had attended music therapy groups (Table 5.3):

A study of three music therapists' experiences of working in inpatient psychiatry found that many worked within a single-session model, with 'working in the moment' being a strong theme. They also reflected on the ways in which they use

Table 5.3 Patient experiences of inpatient music therapy

Release of stress	Healing balm	Concentration	Safe space
Shared experience	Mutual desire for support	Intrinsic value of music	Music learning
Coping with here and now	Motivation/hope	Connection to others	Self-awareness
Lessons for the future	Value of listening and trust	Self-expression	Negative experiences

music to achieve a connection with patients [156]. Finally, a mixed methods PhD study found that offering increased frequency of group music therapy (2–4 times per week) on psychiatric wards was acceptable to in-patients and identified three core processes based on video observation, patient and therapist interviews: engagement; emotional expression and social connection. Active music-making, synchrony and singing were important for group cohesion [157]. Finally, a recent study performed in an acute inward psychiatric context proved that a bi-weekly protocol of active music therapy was able to induce an amelioration of affective symptomatology in patients with psychosis, also in emergency settings [158].

5.5 Future Directions

Despite extensive literature, much more is to be done to understand the processes and build a firmer evidence base for music therapy in psychiatry. As models and methods of music therapy change with current advances in the field, further studies are required to better understand which forms of music therapy 'work best' and 'for whom'. Whilst randomised controlled trials are the pinnacle of providing evidence for effectiveness, the design is especially challenging given the adaptability and complexity of music therapy and range of diagnoses and needs encountered. Outcomes of music therapy are broader than symptomatic relief and more work is required to define and (where applicable) reliably measure and track both the immediate and longer term impact of its benefits and potential harms.

Current trends suggest a move towards recovery and community based work, multi-modal approaches (working across or combining different art forms) and work that goes beyond single diagnoses. For example, the ERA trial is currently testing the effectiveness of three different forms of arts therapy (art, dance movement and music therapy) for diagnostically heterogeneous community patients in a manualised format that highlights the importance of recovery and reconnection to community arts participation as a part of this. There is a striking under-representation of research for some diagnoses (especially anxiety, bipolar and personality disorders), although many are represented in populations of diagnostically heterogeneous studies. In contrast, there are increasing numbers of modifications to the Bonny Method of GIM, many of which are with psychiatric populations. Further areas where there is ongoing research are dementia and carers and perinatal psychiatry, with many large-scale international collaborations.

Moving forward in mental health care, to truly demonstrate the value of music therapy, community music, arts therapies and arts in health, there is more to do than trials alone. There is a need to educate stakeholders as to the spectrum of practice, how this contributes at different stages of recovery, explain the levels of evidence for each and justify when such levels may not be appropriate. There is also a need to conduct further research that supports innovation and development of practice within continuously evolving health contexts. This includes in-depth examination of micro-level processes and relationships. Such questions require high-quality, context-specific qualitative approaches. Multiple types of evidence (especially high-quality qualitative and practice-based enquiry) should be used at a level commensurate with the scale of provision being assessed. Across all evidence—trials or service evaluations, there is a need to ensure the highest quality and rigour. This means transparency about methods of data collection, ensuring viewpoints from multiple stakeholders are represented, minimising bias and ensuring replicability of both the intervention and the evaluation methods.

Values of equality, relationships, creativity and community are at the heart of music therapy. Whatever evidence is collected, the research must remain client-led and take a shared journey. Our clients are not subjects but partners with considerable expertise in their own values, experience and preferences. Working jointly to understand, develop, evidence and share music therapy practice has the best potential to communicate the value of music to stakeholders and how it may benefit society as a whole.

References

1. Tyler H. The music therapy profession in modern Britain. In: Music as medicine: the history of music therapy since antiquity. Aldershot: Ashgate Publishers; 2000.
2. Kern P. World Federation of Music Therapy. 2011. https://www.wfmt.info/2011/05/01/announcing-wfmts-new-definition-of-music-therapy/.
3. Odell-Miller H. The development of clinical music therapy in adult mental health practice: music, health and therapy. In: Medicine, health and the arts: approaches to the medical humanities. London: Routledge; 2014. p. 264–80.
4. McCaffrey T. Music therapy's development in mental healthcare: a historical consideration of early ideas and intersecting agents. Music Med. 2015;7:28–33.
5. Fagin L. A brief narrative history of inpatient care in the United Kingdom. In: Hardcastle M, Kennard D, Grandison S, et al., editors. Experiences of mental health inpatient care. Narratives from service users, carers and professionals. London: Routledge; 2007. p. 8–16.
6. Hardcastle M. Recent times. In: Hardcastle M, Kennard D, Grandison S, et al., editors. Experiences of mental health inpatient care. Narratives from service users, carers and professionals. London: Routledge; 2007. p. 17–20.
7. Bothwell LE, Podolsky SH. The emergence of the randomized, controlled trial. N Engl J Med. 2016;375:501–4.
8. Alvin J. Music therapy. London: Stainer and Bell; 1966.
9. Priestley M. Music therapy in action. Oxford: St Martin's; 1975.
10. Priestley M. Essays on analytical music therapy. Phoenixville, PA: Barcelona Publishers; 1994.
11. Magee M. Music technology in therapeutic and health settings. London: Jessica Kingsley; 2014.

12. Sadnovik N. The birth of a therapeutic recording studio: addressing the needs of the hip-hop generation on an adult psychiatric inpatient unit. In: Music technology in therapeutic and health setting. London: Jessica Kingsley; 2014. p. 247–62.
13. Colbert T, Bent C. Working across modalities in the arts therapies. London: Routledge; 2018.
14. Twyford K, Watson T. Integrated team working: music therapy as part of transdisciplinary and collaborative approaches. London: Jessica Kingsley; 2008.
15. Melhuish R. 'Let them bring their own song': a qualitative study of developing relationships between care staff and nursing home residents with dementia through music therapy and dance movement therapy groups. In: Collaboration and assistance in music therapy practice. London: Jessica Kingsley; 2017. p. 99–119.
16. Odell-Miller H. Exploring the significance of the role of assistants in music therapy groups in adult and older people's mental health settings. In: Collaboration and assistance in music therapy practice. London: Jessica Kingsley; 2017. p. 88–98.
17. Storie S. Group music therapy in a mental health service with older adults: 'it sure beats watching television'. In: Arts therapists in multidisciplinary settings: working together for better outcomes. London: Jessica Kingsley; 2016. p. 109–22.
18. Edwards J. Approaches and models of music therapy. In: The Oxford handbook of music therapy. Oxford, Oxford University Press; 2016. Epub ahead of print 2016. https://doi.org/10.1093/oxfordhb/9780199639755.013.38.
19. Rogers CR. A current formulation of client-centred therapy. Soc Serv Rev. 1950;24:442–8.
20. Odell-Miller H. Are words enough? Music therapy as an influence in psychoanalytic psychotherapy. In: The future of psychoanalytic psychotherapy. London: Whurr Publishers; 2003. p. 153–66.
21. Winnicott DW. Playing and reality. London: Tavisock Publications; 1971. Epub ahead of print 1971. https://doi.org/10.4324/9780429478352.
22. Silverman MJ. Effects of educational music therapy on illness management knowledge and mood state in acute psychiatric inpatients: a randomized three group effectiveness study. Nord J Music Ther. 2016;25:57–75.
23. Silverman MJ. Effects of family-based educational music therapy on acute care psychiatric patients and their family members: an exploratory mixed-methods study. Nord J Music Ther. 2014;23:99–122.
24. Aigen K. Music-centered dimensions of Nordoff-Robbins music therapy. Music Ther Perspect. 2014;32:18–29.
25. Pavlicevic M, Ansdell G, Procter S, et al. Presenting the evidence. Nurs Stand. 2009. Epub ahead of print 2009.; https://doi.org/10.7748/ns.7.3.18.s34.
26. Hannibal N, Schwantes M. Mentalization based treatment (MBT): a possible theoretical frame for music therapy practice in clinical psychiatry. Voices. 2017;17:1–13.
27. Compton DS. A feasibility trial of group cognitive analytic music therapy in secure hospital settings. Cambridge: Anglia Ruskin University; 2014.
28. Compton DS. Beyond body, beyond words: cognitive analytic music therapy in disordered offenders. Music Ther Today. 2006;VII:839–75.
29. Rappaport L. Mindfulness and the arts therapies: theory and practice. London: Jessica Kingsley; 2014.
30. Trondalen G. Relational music therapy: an intersubjective experience. Dallas: Barcelona Publishers; 2016.
31. Trondalen G. Musical intersubjectivity. Arts Psychother. 2019:101589.
32. Rolvsjord R. Resource oriented music therapy in mental health care. Gilsum: Barcelona Publishers; 2014.
33. McCaffrey T, Carr CE, Solli HP, et al. Music therapy and recovery in mental health: seeking a way forward. Voices. Epub ahead of print 2018. https://doi.org/10.15845/voices.v18i1.918.
34. Leamy M, Bird V, Le Boutillier C, et al. Conceptual framework for personal recovery in mental health: systematic review and narrative synthesis. Br J Psychiatry. 2011;199:445–52.
35. Wampold B, Imel ZE. The great psychotherapy debate. 2nd ed. New York: Routledge; 2015.

36. Trevarthen C, Stephen NM. The dance of wellbeing: defining the musical therapeutic effect. Nord Tidsskr Musikkter. 2000;9:4–17.
37. Trondalen G, Skårderud F. Playing with affects: and the importance of "affect attunement". Nord J Music Ther. 2007;16:100–11.
38. Procter S. Reparative musicing: thinking on the usefulness of social capital theory within music therapy. Nord J Music Ther. 2011;20:242–62.
39. Procter S. Playing politics: community music therapy and the therapeutic redistribution of musical capital for mental health. In: Pavlicevic M, Ansdell G, editors. Community music therapy. London: Jessica Kingsley; 2004. p. 214–30.
40. Procter S. Empowering and enabling. Voices. 2001;1 https://doi.org/10.15845/voices.v1i2.58.
41. Pedersen IN. Music therapy in psychiatry today - do we need specialization based on the reduction of diagnosis-specific symptoms or on the overall development of patients' resources? Or do we need both? Nord J Music Ther. 2014;23:173–94.
42. De Backer J. Music and psychosis: a research report detailing the transition from sensorial play to musical form by psychotic patients. Nord J Music Ther. 2008;17:89–104.
43. Tostmann J, Metzner S. Ko-kreative Momente und Transition: Eine qualitative Studie zu Abstimmungsprozessen in der musiktherapeutischen Psychosenbehandlung. Music Umschau. 2017;38:356–66.
44. Gold C, Mössler K, Grocke D, et al. Individual music therapy for mental health care clients with low therapy motivation: multicentre randomised controlled trial. Psychother Psychosom. 2013;82:319–31.
45. Grocke D, Bloch S, Castle D, et al. Group music therapy for severe mental illness: a randomized embedded-experimental mixed methods study. Acta Psychiatr Scand. 2014;130:144–53.
46. Chanda ML, Levitin DJ. The neurochemistry of music. Trends Cogn Sci. 2013;17:179–93.
47. Tarr B, Launay J, Dunbar RIM. Music and social bonding: 'self-other' merging and neurohormonal mechanisms. Front Psychol. 2014;5:1–10.
48. Dunbar RIM, Kaskatis K, MacDonald I, et al. Performance of music elevates pain threshold and positive affect: implications for the evolutionary function of music. Evol Psychol. 2012;10:688–702.
49. Weinstein D, Launay J, Pearce E, et al. Singing and social bonding: changes in connectivity and pain threshold as a function of group size. Evol Hum Behav. 2016;37:152–8.
50. Ansdell G. How music helps in music therapy and every day life. Farnham: Ashgate Publishers; 2014.
51. De Nora T. Music asylums: wellbeing through music in everyday life. Farnham: Ashgate Publishers; 2015.
52. Ansdell G, Davidson J, Magee WL, et al. From 'This F***ing life' to 'that's better'... in four minutes: an interdisciplinary study of music therapy's 'present moments' and their potential for affect modulation. Nord J Music Ther. 2010;19:3–28.
53. Rolvsjord R. What clients do to make music therapy work: a qualitative multiple case study in adult mental health care. Nord J Music Ther. 2015;24:296–321.
54. Carr C, Odell-Miller H, Priebe S. A systematic review of music therapy practice and outcomes with acute adult psychiatric in-patients. PLoS One. 8. Epub ahead of print 2013. https://doi.org/10.1371/journal.pone.0070252.
55. Bonny H, Savary L. Music and your mind: listening with a new consciousness. Barcelona: Barcelona Publishers; 1973.
56. Booth JM. Music, drawing and narrative: an adaptation of the Bonny method of guided imagery and music. J Assoc Music Imag. 10
57. Pilling S, Anderson I, Goldberg D, et al. Guidelines: depression in adults, including those with a chronic physical health problem: summary of NICE guidance. BMJ. 2009;339:1025–7.
58. Goldberg F. The Bonny method of guided imagery and music as individual and group treatment in a Short-trem acute psychiatric hospital. J Assoc Music Imag. 1994;3:18–34.
59. Moe T. Group guided imagery and music therapy for inpatients with substance abuse disorder. J Assoc Music Imag. 2011;13:77–98.

60. Murphy KM, Ziedonis DM. Group guided imagery and music for adults in addiction treatment: a pilot randomized controlled trial feasibly study. J Assoc Music Imag. 2016;16:43–65.
61. Summer L. Group music and imagery therapy: emergent receptive techniques in music therapy practice. In: Bruscia KE, Grocke D, editors. Guided imagery and music: the Bonny method and beyond. Gilsum: Barcelona Publishers; 2002.
62. Wrangsjö B, Körlin D. Guided imagery and music (GIM) as a psychotherapeutic method in psychiatry. 1995.
63. Körlin D. Music breathing breath grounding and modulation of the Bonyn method of guided imagery and music (BMGIM). J Assoc Music Imag. 2007;11:79–109.
64. Silverman MJ. The effect of single-session psychoeducational music therapy on verbalizations and perceptions in psychiatric patients. J Music Ther. 2009;46:105–31.
65. Silverman MJ. Effects of educational music therapy on state hope for recovery in acute care mental health inpatients: a cluster-randomized effectiveness study. Front Psychol. 2016;7:1–10.
66. Hanser SB, Thompson LW. Effects of a music therapy strategy on depressed older adults. J Gerontol. 1994;49:265–9.
67. Curtis A. Music therapists at Anglia Ruskin aiming to help dementia sufferers with £2.7m project. Cambridge Independent. 2019. https://www.cambridgeindependent.co.uk/news/anglia-ruskin-university-music-therapists-aiming-to-help-dementia-sufferers-with-2-7m-project-9070704/.
68. Wigram T. Improvisation: methods and techniques for music therapy clinicians, educators and students. London: Jessica Kingsley; 2004.
69. Ridder HMO. Singing dialogue: music therapy with persons in advanced stages of dementia. Denmark: Aalborg University; 2003.
70. Dassa A, Amir D. The role of singing familiar songs in encouraging conversation among people with middle to late stage alzheimer's disease. J Music Ther. 2014;51:131–53.
71. Baker FA, Wigram T, Stott D, et al. Therapeutic songwriting in music therapy: Part I: Who are the therapists, who are the clients, and why is songwriting used? Nord J Music Ther. 2008;17:105–23.
72. Day T, Baker FA, Darlington Y. Beyond the therapy room: women's experiences of 'going public' with song creations. Br J Music Ther. 2016;23:19–26.
73. McCaffrey T, Edwards J. 'Music therapy helped me get back doing': perspectives of music therapy participants in mental health services. J Music Ther. 2016;53:121–48.
74. Baker FA, Wigram T, Stott D, et al. Therapeutic songwriting in music therapy. Part II: Comparing the literature with practice across diverse clinical populations. Nord J Music Ther. 2009;18:32–56.
75. Windle E, Hickling LM, Jayacodi S, et al. The experiences of patients in the synchrony group music therapy trial for long-term depression. Arts Psychother. Epub ahead of print. 2019; https://doi.org/10.1016/j.aip.2019.101580.
76. Silverman MJ. Effects of group songwriting on motivation and readiness for treatment on patients in detoxification: a randomized wait-list effectiveness study. J Music Ther. 2012;49:414–29.
77. Silverman MJ. Effects of group-based educational songwriting on craving in patients on a detoxification unit: a cluster-randomized effectiveness study. Psychol Music. 2019;47:241–54.
78. Aasgaard T, Blichfeldt Ærø SC. Songwriting techniques in music therapy practice. In: Edwards J, editor. The Oxford handbook of music therapy. Oxford, Oxford University Press. p. 1–33.
79. Odell-Miller H. The practice of music therapy for adults with mental health problems: the relationship between diagnosis and clinical method Odell-Miller, Helen. In: The practice of music therapy for adults with mental health problems: the relationship. Denmark: Aalborg University; 2007.
80. Geretsegger M, Ka M, Xj C, et al. Music therapy for people with schizophrenia and schizophrenia-like disorders. Cochrane Database Syst Rev. 2017;5(5):CD004025. https://doi.org/10.1002/14651858.CD004025.pub4.

81. Metzner S, Jaeger U, Masuhr O, et al. Forms of attunement during the initial stages of music therapy for patients with acute psychosis – a multicentre clinical study. Nord J Music Ther. 2018;27:360–80.
82. Kosugi N, Oshiyama C, Kodama N, et al. Incorporating music therapy into cognitive remediation to improve both cognitive dysfunction and negative symptoms in schizophrenia. Schizophr Res. 2019;204:423–4.
83. Solli HP, Rolvsjord R. "The opposite of treatment": a qualitative study of how patients diagnosed with psychosis experience music therapy. Nord J Music Ther. 2015;24:67–92.
84. Solli HP. "Shut up and play!": improvisational use of popular music for a man with schizophrenia. Nord J Music Ther. 2008;17:67–77.
85. Gavrielidou M, Odell-Miller H. An investigation of pivotal moments in music therapy in adult mental health. Arts Psychother. 2017;52:50–62.
86. Moe T, Roesen A, Raben H. Restitutional factors in group music therapy with psychiatric patients based on a modification of guided imagery and music (Gim). Nord Tidsskr Musikkter. 2000;9:36–50.
87. Maratos A, Crawford MJ, Procter S, et al. Music therapy for depression: it seems to work, but how? Br J Psychiatry. 2011;199:92–3.
88. Aalbers S, Fusar-Poli L, Freeman RE, et al. Music therapy for depression. Cochrane Database Syst Rev. Epub ahead of print. 2017; https://doi.org/10.1002/14651858.CD004517.pub3.
89. Zhao K, Bai ZG, Bo A, et al. A systematic review and meta-analysis of music therapy for the older adults with depression. Int J Geriatr Psychiatry. 2016;31:1188–98.
90. Trimmer C, Tyo R, Pikard J, et al. Low-intensity cognitive behavioural therapy-based music group (CBT-music) for the treatment of symptoms of anxiety and depression: a feasibility study. Behav Cogn Psychother. 2018;46:168–81.
91. Zarate R. Clinical improvisation and its effect on anxiety: a multiple single subject design. Arts Psychother. 2016;48:46–53.
92. Gutiérrez EOF, Camarena VAT. Music therapy in generalized anxiety disorder. Arts Psychother. 2015;44:19–24.
93. Shirani Bidabadi S, Mehryar A. Music therapy as an adjunct to standard treatment for obsessive compulsive disorder and co-morbid anxiety and depression: a randomized clinical trial. J Affect Disord. 2015;184:13–7.
94. Chang YS, Chu H, Yang CY, et al. The efficacy of music therapy for people with dementia: a meta-analysis of randomised controlled trials. J Clin Nurs. 2015;24:3425–40.
95. Ueda T, Suzukamo Y, Sato M, et al. Effects of music therapy on behavioral and psychological symptoms of dementia: a systematic review and meta-analysis. Ageing Res Rev. 2013;12:628–41.
96. Raglio A, Bellelli G, Traficante D, et al. Efficacy of music therapy in the treatment of behavioural and psychiatric symptoms of dementia. Alzheimer Dis Assoc Disord. 2008; 22:158–62.
97. Raglio A, Bellelli G, Traficante D, et al. Efficacy of music therapy treatment based on cycles of sessions: a randomised controlled trial. Aging Ment Heal. 2010;14:900–4.
98. Raglio A, Bellandi D, Baiardi P, et al. Effect of active music therapy and individualized listening to music on dementia: a multicenter randomized controlled trial. J Am Geriatr Soc. 2015;63:1534–9.
99. Thornley J, Hirjee H, Vasudev A. Music therapy in patients with dementia and behavioral disturbance on an inpatient psychiatry unit: results from a pilot randomized controlled study. Int Psychogeriatr. 2016;28:869–71.
100. Ridder HMO, Stige B, Qvale LG, et al. Individual music therapy for agitation in dementia: an exploratory randomized controlled trial. Aging Ment Health. 2013;17:667–78.
101. Hsu MH, Flowerdew R, Parker M, et al. Individual music therapy for managing neuropsychiatric symptoms for people with dementia and their carers: a cluster randomised controlled feasibility study. BMC Geriatr. 2015;15:1–19.
102. McDermott O, Orrell M, Ridder HM. The development of music in dementia assessment scales (MiDAS). Nord J Music Ther. 2015;24:232–51.

103. McDermott O, Orgeta V, Ridder HM, et al. A preliminary psychometric evaluation of music in dementia assessment scales (MiDAS). Int Psychogeriatr. 2014;26:1011–9.
104. Schall A, Haberstroh J, Pantel J. Time series analysis of individual music therapy in dementia: effects on communication behavior and emotionalwell-being. GeroPsych. 2015;28:113–22.
105. Baker FA, Bloska J, Braat S, et al. HOMESIDE: home-based family delivered music and reading interventions for people living with dementia: protocol of a randomised controlled trial. BMJ Open. 2019;9(11):e031332.
106. Floen SK, Elklit A. Psychiatric diagnoses, trauma, and suicidiality. Ann General Psychiatry. 2007;6:1–8.
107. Bryson SA, Gauvin E, Jamieson A, et al. What are effective strategies for implementing trauma-informed care in youth inpatient psychiatric and residential treatment settings? A realist systematic review. Int J Ment Health Syst. 2017;11:1–16.
108. Fazel M, Wheeler J, Danesh J. Prevalence of serious mental disorder in 7000 refugees resettled in. Lancet. 2005;365:1309–14.
109. Richardson LK, Frueh BC, Acierno R. Prevalence estimates of combat-related post-traumatic stress disorder: critical review. Aust N Z J Psychiatry. 2010;44:4–19.
110. Baker FA, Metcalf O, Varker T, et al. A systematic review of the efficacy of creative arts therapies in the treatment of adults with PTSD. Psychol Trauma Theory Res Pract Policy. 2018;10:643–51.
111. Carr CE, D'Ardenne P, Sloboda A, et al. Group music therapy for patients with persistent post-traumatic stress disorder – an exploratory randomized controlled trial with mixed methods evaluation. Psychol Psychother Theory Res Pract. 2012;85:179–202.
112. Jespersen KV, Vuust P. The effect of relaxation music listening on sleep quality in traumatized refugees: a pilot study. J Music Ther. 2012;49:205–29.
113. Landis-Shack N, Heinz AJ, Bonn-Miller MO. Music therapy for posttraumatic stress in adults: a theoretical review. Psychomusicology. 2017;27:334–42.
114. Blake RL. Vietnam veterans with post traumatic stress disorder: findings from a music and imagery project.
115. Sutton J, De Backer J. Music, trauma and silence: the state of the art. Arts Psychother. 2009;36:75–83.
116. Bensimon M, Amir D, Wolf Y. Drumming through trauma: music therapy with post-traumatic soldiers. Arts Psychother. 2008;35:34–48.
117. Beck BD, Messel C, Meyer SL, et al. Feasibility of trauma-focused guided imagery and music with adult refugees diagnosed with PTSD: a pilot study. Nord J Music Ther. 2018;27:67–86.
118. Maack C. Outcomes and processes of the Bonny method of guided imagery and music (GIM) and its adaptations and psychodynamic imaginative trauma therapy (PITT) for women with complex PTSD. Denmark: Aalborg University; 2012.
119. Smeijsters H. Music therapy with anorexia nervosa: an integrative theoretical and methodological perspective. Thousand Oaks: Sage Publicatons; 1993. p. 3–13.
120. Robarts JZ, Sloboda A. Perspectives on music therapy with people suffering from anorexia nervosa. J Br Music Ther. 1994;8:7–14.
121. Bibb J, Castle D, Newton R. The role of music therapy in reducing post meal related anxiety for patients with anorexia nervosa. J Eat Disord. 2015;3:1–6.
122. Lejonclou A, Trondalen G. I've started to move into my own body: music therapy with women suffering from eating disorders. Nord J Music Ther. 2009;18:79–92.
123. Frisch MJ, Franko DL, Herzog DB. Arts-based therapies in the treatment of eating disorders. Eat Disord. 2006;14:131–42.
124. Bateman A, Fonagy P. Mentalization based treatment for borderline personality disorder. World Psychiatry. 2010;9:11–5.
125. Strehlow G, Hannibal N. Mentalizing in improvisational music therapy. Nord J Music Ther. 2019;28:333–46.
126. Hannibal N, Nygaard Pedersen I, Bonde LO, et al. A pilot study investigating research design feasibility using pre-post measures to test the effect of music therapy in psychiatry with people diagnosed with personality disorders. Voices. 2019;19:1–19.

127. Pool J, Odell-Miller H. Aggression in music therapy and its role in creativity with reference to personality disorder. Arts Psychother. 2011;38:169–77.
128. Strehlow G, Lindner R. Music therapy interaction patterns in relation to borderline personality disorder (BPD) patients. Nord J Music Ther. 2016;25:134–58.
129. Short H. It feels like Armageddon: identification with a female personality-disordered offender at a time of cultural, political and personal attack. Nord J Music Ther. 2017;26:272–85.
130. Hohmann L, Bradt J, Stegemann T, et al. Effects of music therapy and music-based interventions in the treatment of substance use disorders: A systematic review. PLoS One. 2017. Epub ahead of print 2017.; https://doi.org/10.1371/journal.pone.0187363.
131. Megranahan K, Lynskey MT. Do creative arts therapies reduce substance misuse? A systematic review. Arts Psychother. 2018;57:50–8.
132. Gardstrom SC, Bartkowski J, Willenbrink J, et al. The impact of group music therapy on negative affect of people with co-occurring substance use disorders mental illnesses. Music Ther Perspect. 2013;31:116–26.
133. World Health Organisation. Maternal, newborn, child and adolescent health. https://www.who.int/maternal_child_adolescent/topics/maternal/maternal_perinatal/en/.
134. NHS England. Perinatal. https://www.england.nhs.uk/mental-health/perinatal/.
135. Mastnak W. Perinatal music therapy and antenatal music classes: principles, mechanisms, and benefits. J Perinat Educ. 2016;25:184–92.
136. Friedman SH, Kaplan RS, Rosenthal MB, et al. Music therapy in perinatal psychiatry: use of lullabies for pregnant and postpartum women with mental illness. Music Med. 2010;2:219–25.
137. Chen XJ, Leith H, Aarø LE, et al. Music therapy for improving mental health problems of offenders in correctional settings: systematic review and meta-analysis. J Exp Criminol. 2016;12:209–28.
138. Loth H. Music therapy and forensic psychiatry—choice, denial and the law. J Br Music Ther. 1994;8:10–8.
139. Hakvoort L. Rap music therapy in forensic psychiatry: emphasis on the musical approach to rap. Music Ther Perspect. 2015;33:184–92.
140. Gold C, Voracek M, Wigram T. Effects of music therapy for children and adolescents with psychopathology: a meta-analysis. J Child Psychol Psychiatry Allied Discip. 2004;45:1054–63.
141. Goldbeck L, Ellerkamp T. A randomized controlled trial of multimodal music therapy for children with anxiety disorders. J Music Ther. 2012;49:395–413.
142. Shuman J, Kennedy H, DeWitt P, et al. Group music therapy impacts mood states of adolescents in a psychiatric hospital setting. Arts Psychother. 2016;49:50–6.
143. Porter S, McConnell T, McLaughlin K, et al. Music therapy for children and adolescents with behavioural and emotional problems: a randomised controlled trial. J Child Psychol Psychiatry Allied Discip. 2017;58:586–94.
144. Oldfield A, Bell K, Pool J. Three families and three music therapists: reflections on short term music therapy in child and family psychiatry. Nord J Music Ther. 2012;21:250–67.
145. Suetani S, Batterham M. Un-rapping teen spirit: use of rap music as a treatment tool in adolescence psychiatry. Aust N Z J Psychiatry. 2015;49:670.
146. Preyde M, Berends A, Parehk S, et al. Adolescents' evaluation of music therapy in an inpatient psychiatric unit: a quality improvement project. Music Ther Perspect. 2017;35:58–62.
147. Silverman MJ. Effects of music therapy on psychiatric patients' proactive coping skills: two pilot studies. Arts Psychother. 2011;38:125–9.
148. Iliya YA. Singing for healing and hope: music therapy methods that use the voice with individuals who are homeless and mentally ill. Music Ther Perspect. 2011;29:14–22.
149. Silverman MJ, Baker FA, MacDonald RAR. Flow and meaningfulness as predictors of therapeutic outcome within songwriting interventions. Psychol Music. 2016;44:1331–45.
150. Baker FA, Silverman MJ, MacDonald R. Reliability and validity of the meaningfulness of songwriting scale (MSS) with adults on acute psychiatric and detoxification units. J Music Ther. 2016;53:55–74.
151. Degli Stefani M, Biasutti M. Effects of music therapy on drug therapy of adult psychiatric outpatients: a pilot randomized controlled study. Front Psychol. 2016;7:1–8.

152. Silverman MJ. Effects of a live educational music therapy intervention on acute psychiatric inpatients' perceived social support and trust in the therapist: a four-group randomized effectiveness study. J Music Ther. 2015;51:228–49.
153. Markovich R, Tatsumi K. The effects of single-session music therapy interventions in comparison with a cognitive behavioral intervention on mood with adult psychiatric inpatients in an acute-care setting: a quasi-experimental trial. Music Ther Perspect. 2015;33:118–27.
154. Deatrich KG, Prout MF, Boyer BA, et al. Effectiveness of group music therapy in a psychiatric hospital: a randomized pilot study of treatment outcome. Int J Group Psychother. 2016;66:592–617.
155. MacDonald S. Client experiences in music therapy in the psychiatric inpatient milieu. Music Ther Perspect. 2015;33:108–17.
156. Chen YY. Single-session improvisational group music therapy in adult inpatient psychiatry: a pilot study of the therapist's experience. Nord J Music Ther. 2019;28:151–68.
157. Carr C. Modelling of intensive group music therapy for acute adult psychiatric inpatients. PhD Thesis. Queen Mary University, 2014.
158. Volpe U, Gianoglio C, Autiero L, Marino ML, Facchini D, Mucci A, Galderisi S. Acute Effects of Music Therapy in Subjects With Psychosis During Inpatient Treatment. Psychiatry. 2018;81(3):218–27.

From an Empirical Approach to Scientific Evidence: Reflections on Music Therapy and Psychiatry

6

Gabriela Wagner

This chapter written by Emma Windle and Catherine Carr provides a brief, but yet careful and elaborated overview on music therapy (MT) in the field of mental health covering topics as history of clinical practice, underpinned theories, basic principles and techniques, research and future challenges in western culture. There is a wide bibliographic reference available for the reader interested in further information on the abovementioned issues.

When reading the reviewed scientific evidence, several questions emerged in the light of practical experience in the field of music therapy. First, one may consider what are the main contributions of this chapter to understand the multifaceted sound/music-human being-sound/music [1] complex relationship? And why is the practice of intentional use of musical experience considered efficient in the treatment of emotional disorders since remote times? How does the evidence-based MT benefit every day in clinical practice? How does research contribute to professional image of music therapists? What are the possible biases in evidence-based MT, a very precious path for music therapists in their academic training? And finally, what is music in a music therapy process? Is it nothing but organized noises? [2]. Is it possible to extract music from the context of a significant therapeutic relationship where its value is singular and unique as a mediator of communication?

We agree with those who consider that music is characterized both by its ubiquity and its antiquity [3]. There is no doubt about the fact that the history of music therapy therefore the intentional use of music in psychiatry has passed through different stages. It is also clear that the empirical approach of the Fifties and Seventies became into a clinical practice based on scientific evidence in a great variety of fields of clinical practice in western culture.

G. Wagner (✉)
Universidad del Salvador, Buenos Aires, Argentina

Mental Health Department, Hospital de Clínicas, José de San Martín, Buenos Aires, Argentina

U. Volpe (ed.), *Arts Therapies in Psychiatric Rehabilitation*, https://doi.org/10.1007/978-3-030-76208-7_6

In the second half of the twentieth century, there has been a great take-off of the pharmaceutical industry in psychiatry. The successive discoveries of new medications with activity in the sphere of human behavior allowed the outpatient treatments in mental health care, reducing the time of hospitalization. The adequate treatment of these psychiatric patients demanded new attention devices. Day hospitals quickly spread out offering new approaches for treatment. MT, and in general art therapy, became important options. In the early Seventies, the development of new technology for manipulating sounds, noises, and music facilitated recording, transporting, and analyzing the sonorous-musical interaction of music therapy sessions. These achievements allowed taking the first steps in scientific research in music therapy. At the same time, the entry and diffusion of electronic music caused a definite revolution of the concept of music.

When designing a research on MT effects in psychiatric patients, it is important to consider that without a family or support group, regular medication and an adequate treatment there is an increase of the relapse risk. This tripod is the complex support of the treatment. It is difficult to isolate any of these variables in order to be able to detect specific art/music therapy effects in mental health treatment processes.

As regarding to professional identity other questions emerge. Are people involved in the field of MT music therapists, sound therapist, or sound/music therapists? How do we define music? The term "music therapy" refers simultaneously to two interrelated fields of inquiry. On the one hand, the expression is used to make reference to a scientific discipline whose object of study is the complex of sound-human being-sound, as well as the search for diagnostic elements and derived therapeutic methods. On the other hand, the same term is used to define specific process and procedures attempting to modify psychodynamic aspects of the personality and to overcome pathological symptoms [4].

With this personal reflection I would like to focus on one of the biases on evidence-based MT, which lies in the definition of MT itself. What is the role of music in the acoustic scene of a music therapy session? What are the aesthetic criteria when we talk about music? What is its semiotics? Should we include both spoken and sang language, unorganized instrumental sequences, or infinite silences? Cultural aspects should be also considered as a possible bias element in mental health assessment. For instance, certain type of "consultations" to spiritual entities described by original people of Argentina during professional evaluations out of cultural context can be understood as delirium. Anthropological issues are essential to distinguish a delusion from a spiritual community construction of shared beliefs or myths, as shown in a clinical case reported in Table 6.1.

Music is an expression of culture and it can be affected by a countless number of factors.

Table 6.1 A clinical case of culturally informed MT

Miguel was a 28-year-old man who was brought to the hospital's emergency room by the police. He was found at night running and screaming unintelligible words addressed to an invisible person. Some of the most recurring words were "God, devil, witches, spirits and hell." His symptoms fitted with mystical delusion with psychotic outbreak and M. was hospitalized with a diagnosis of schizophrenia
M. was raised up by his grandmother in a small bilingual community at Northwest of Argentina. After they were abandoned by Miguel's father, his mother came to work to Buenos Aires in order to be able to maintain her two children and her mother. The first language he learned was Quechua and later Spanish. He was 18 when he came to Buenos Aires to live with her mother. M. had two girls. He didn't live with them and their mother, but collaborated in their maintenance. He worked as a wall painter, but he couldn't find any job. As his condition deteriorated, he stopped visiting them
After his crisis was over, he was treated as an outpatient by an interdisciplinary team in the day hospital. Among other milieu therapies he had weekly group music therapy for 6 months. Although M. spoke Spanish, he couldn't get integrated in group or individual psychotherapy. He was referred to additional individual music therapy sessions because of his interest in becoming a folk singer. Unfortunately, he didn't have a fine tuned voice neither the coordination for singing and playing the guitar at the same time
As part of his treatment each sonorous-musical activity was recorded and used as an "auditory mirror" for self-recognition and to distinguish inner and outer voices. The techniques were reconstructive, analytically and catharsis oriented with an emphasis on insight and support. There is no space for more details, but it's important to comment that with a few simple folk chords, as a troubadour of his soul he shared his inner world composing recitation songs
Improvising by sounding up his childhood we could find out about not only the extreme poverty in which he grew up but also the everyday life and traditions of his community. We could learn about Salamanca, or Sall o Salla-folk musicians gathering, Mancca-down, that means deepness. Salamanca is a space dedicated to teaching and to the exchange of knowledge located 50 m deep in the mountains where the initiates learn the art that interests him (games, dance, play the guitar, heal and bother others) thanks to Supay, the devil. The tradition says if someone listened to his music, he would have a life of terror, unless the prayers a person of good faith helped him not to fall into his temptation. Talking with these spirits was usual in this cultural syncretism where music was a temptation, a pleasure, and a motivation to get lost. From his point of view, the music therapist was this person with good faith
His verbal expression improved. For a better outcome his diagnosis had to be changed as well as his medication
A week before his discharge he told to his psychiatrist that he couldn't help to consult Salamanca again. There was an unjustified fear of a new crisis. In his community lying is not natural. He needed the advice to calculate the profit for his work. He knew the cost of his effort and of the materials he needed to buy, but the profit was a trick-like addition that was not entirely honest to him
In this case, the symptoms fitted with mystical delusion with psychotic outbreak were not a disturbance in relationship to the external world or in the sense of self, but the result of a cultural background. He was discharged from the hospital, but returns to ask for help and advice when he finds it necessary. M. is in touch with his children, works as a wall painter and learns guitar

Windle and Carr focus their attention on the effects of musical experience and analyze relevant evidence-based researches linking results with many issues faced by clients living with mental illness across different stages and life courses. There is methodic analysis of relevant evidence-based MT papers in 12 different mental health areas. As about the conduction of these processes by professional music therapists and other health crisis workers with a musical background may assume this role. The question is what is the incidence of specific professional training on the effectiveness of a music therapy process. Regarding this matter, there are often crucial differences. With reference to the specificity, in Argentina there are several university careers and there is a National of Music Therapy Law approved in 2015 by the Senate and the Chamber of Deputies of the National Congress to regulate its professional practice [5].

The future directions proposed by the review are highly motivating for new researches. The authors mention an interesting question related with the abovementioned issues about music and art therapist's professional profile. "What makes us the same and what makes as different?" An original ongoing ERA (European Research Area) study designed as an NIHR (National Institute for Health Research) funded, multicoated, randomized, controlled trial of groups' arts therapies compared to group counseling in community mental health care, focused on the volunteered service users and the different therapists' dynamic interaction process and effectiveness.

This study published in this book shares a great amount of information which contributes to the building of knowledge in MT and it demonstrates a deep knowledge in research methods and reflects remarkable and interesting professional career.

The above reflections and comments on MT and psychiatry may lead us to new fields of practice, and of course new questions and research. For example, the increased scope of telehealth MT and Arts Therapy since the onset of the pandemic demands new research to establish wider relationships of benefits and challenges in the process of transition from in-person (pre-COVID 19) to telehealth service (since COVID-19) for psychiatric patients. There is a need to reconsider recommendation, and demand criteria, techniques, tools, procedures and effectiveness in these fields. These innovated clinical routes await research and confirmation with structural studies.

References

1. Benenzon R. Manual de Musicoterapia. Buenos Aires, Barcelona: Paidós; 1981.
2. Monsergas Carceller J. Introducción y comentario a Hyperprism de Edgard Varése. Balencia: Institució Alfons el Magnànim; 2017.
3. Huron D. Voice leading: the science behind a musical art. MA: MIT Press; 2016.
4. Wagner G. A Avaliaçao Neurosonoro-Musical e o tratamiento Musicoterapeutico de Afásico. In: Benenzon R, editor. Contribuçao ao conhecimiento do contexto nao verbal. San Pablo: Summus; 1988.
5. The National Law of Music Therapy Profession 27.153. Boletin official, 3 de Julio 2015, Buenos Aires. 2015.

Professional Flexibility Towards the Clients' Needs in Music Therapy and Music Medicine in Psychiatry

7

Inge Nygaard Pedersen

Having been head of the Music Therapy Clinic—an integrated institution between Aalborg University and Aalborg University Hospital, Psychiatry, Denmark since 1995, it is confirming and encouraging to read this comprehensive overview of evidence-based research in music therapy in psychiatry.

Music therapists in Denmark have increasingly performed RCT and pilot studies for coming RCT studies during the last years [1–3]. The main reason is that the Danish Health System does not allow any treatment to be recommended in the National Guidelines, unless it is proved that international evidence based results are replicable in the Danish Health System. This is a problem for music therapy in psychiatry in Denmark, being a small country with only one music therapy education. Twenty music therapists are currently employed in psychiatry, equally distributed between hospital and social psychiatry.

Danish music therapists are, through comprehensively therapeutic training in the form of self-inquiry, self-experience, and self-development integrated in all 5 years of the full-time BA/MA university music therapy program, specifically trained to be aware of meeting different needs by the clients at different phases in a treatment process. They do not seek or follow a move towards recovery and community based work as a trend or an ideology. They are trained to closely follow the process of the client and to work in depth with psychodynamic forces, when this is appropriate and with resources and recovery, when this is appropriate [4]. As the authors of the review chapter write: "there are many ways in which music therapy can be applied to help support both symptoms and their wider secondary impacts upon people living with mental illness." These authors also state: "A common misconception is that the therapeutic action lies solely within the music itself." In our clinical practice in music therapy in Denmark, we are very aware that the therapist/client relationship

I. N. Pedersen (✉)
Aalborg University, Aalborg, Denmark

Music Therapy Clinic, Aalborg University Hospital, Psychiatry, Aalborg, Denmark
e-mail: innp@rn.dk

U. Volpe (ed.), *Arts Therapies in Psychiatric Rehabilitation*,
https://doi.org/10.1007/978-3-030-76208-7_7

is of outmost importance, and that music improvisation, -listening, and -performing grows out of the quality of the relationship. When music listening is applied without a music therapist being present, we consistently call the activity "music medicine" and not music therapy [5].

In Denmark, music therapy treatment and research in psychiatry have primarily been developed with people suffering from schizophrenia [1] where an RCT blinded study with a control group condition also including music currently is performed. Research has also been performed with people suffering from personality disorders [2] with traumatized refugees [1] in forensic psychiatry [6] and in depression-related insomnia [7]. Concerning the latter, the approach is music listening. Two Danish music therapists have developed an app called The Music Star with many hours of selected playlists. This app is available in a special tablet in aluminum case, equipped with armored glass for safety reasons. The tablet is increasingly installed at client's rooms at many psychiatric hospitals and community units where people suffering from mental health problems are temporarily staying or long time living. The tablet also leaves space for clients' specific music choice [8]. The playlists are chosen from principles of supportive music in a continuum from (1) the supportive and safe field to (2) the supportive and opening field to (3) the supportive and exploring field—following a taxonomy developed by Wärja and Bonde [9].

In the RCT study [2] concerning music therapy as treatment for negative symptoms for people suffering from schizophrenia, we have incorporated a control group activity, where the participants share the same amount of time with a caregiver and are allowed to listen to The Music Star. It is not possible to make any other musical activity and thus not possible to meet the individualized needs of the participants.

We have comprehensive research in the area of dementia, but this is not uniquely classified as music therapy in psychiatry. It is a comprehensive working area for Danish music therapists thanks to professor Ridders research efforts over many years. These efforts are now merging with the efforts of many international colleges in a preparation for a huge multinational cluster-randomized trial [10].

References

1. Beck BD, Lund S, Søgaard U, et al. Music therapy versus treatment as usual for refugees diagnosed with posttraumatic stress disorder (PTSD): study protocol for a randomized controlled trial. Trials. 2018;19:301. https://doi.org/10.1186/s13063-018-2662-z.
2. Pedersen IN, Bonde LO, Nielsen RE, et al. Music therapy as treatment of negative symptoms for adult patients diagnosed with schizophrenia: study protocol for a randomized, controlled and blinded study. Medicines. 2019;6(46):1–15. https://doi.org/10.3390/medicines6020046.
3. Hannibal NJ, Pedersen IN, Bonde LO, et al. A pilot study investigating research design feasibility using pre-post measures to test the effect of music therapy in psychiatry with people diagnosed with personality disorders. Voices. 2019;1:1–19. https://doi.org/10.15845/voices.v19i1.2731.
4. Pedersen IN. Music therapy in psychiatry today – do we need specialization based on the reduction of diagnosis-specific symptoms or on the overall development of patients` resources? Or do we need both? Nord J Music Ther. 2014;23:173–94. https://doi.org/10.1080/08098131.2013.790917.

5. Bonde LO. Five approaches to music as health promotion. Biomed J Sci Tech Res. 2019;15:11349–50. https://doi.org/10.26717/BJSTR.2019.15.002696.
6. Frederiksen B. The development of therapeutic alliance in music therapy with forensic psychiatric patients with schizophrenia. Denmark: Aalborg University; 2019.
7. Lund HN, Pedersen IN, Paaske S, et al. Music to improve sleep quality in adults with depression-related insomnia (MUSTAFI): study protocol for a randomized controlled trial. Trials. 2020;21:305. https://doi.org/10.1186/s13063-020-04247-9.
8. Lund HN, Bertelsen LR, Bonde LO. Sound and music interventions in psychiatry at Aalborg University Hospital. SoundEffects. 2016;6:48–68.
9. Wärja M, Bonde LO. Music as co-therapist: towards a taxanomy of music in therapeutic music and imagery work. Music Med. 2014;6:16–27.
10. Gold C, Assmus J, Stige B, Wake JD, Baker FA, Tamplin J, Clark I, Y-EC L, Jacobsen SL, Ridder HMO, et al. Music interventions for dementia and depression in eLderly care (MIDDEL): protocol and statistical analysis plan for a multinational cluster-randomised trial. BMJ Open. 2019;9(3):e023436. https://doi.org/10.1136/bmjopen-2018-023436.

Music as Central Mechanism for Music Therapy in Mental Health

8

Laurien Hakvoort

Evidence-based MT is developed to ensure that clients receive MT treatment that meets the latest treatment guidelines and incorporate the latest insights in the working mechanisms of MT to meet the most recent understanding of mental functioning and cultural responsivity of the clients. Yet, Coomans [1] concludes in her article on meaningful moments in music therapy, a "review does not lead the reader to one, clear, universal concept that can be transferred to a more general music therapy practice (…). Instead, it provides readers with a comprehensive overview of many different concepts, developed from diverse theoretical backgrounds and clinical contexts."

To make clear choices for a review seems to be extremely hard. An overview of research articles dealing with MT for schizophrenia and psychosis provides an inside in these difficulties. More than 50 articles have been published on MT for patients with psychotic features over the last 2 years, including systematic reviews of the literature [2], qualitative interviews with treatment users [3, 4], reports on stakeholders' perspectives [5], new research protocols [6], randomized controlled researches addressing MT in acute adult psychiatry (e.g., [7, 8]) or in acute care for young populations (e.g., [9, 10]). These studies generally indicate that MT results in decline of negative symptoms, *affirms client's strengths* and *coping skills* and that it can be used as an intervention to *integrate cognitive and affective therapeutic processes* [11]. However, while some articles advise music listening mapped to client's preference [9], others advise specific and very different approaches, ranging from heavy metal [12], through lyric analysis [10], to musical improvisation [8]. To prevent getting overwhelmed by the constantly prompting new research, it might be advisable to limit the information to the last 2 years, avoid research older than 10 years, in the light of the rapid changes in mental health care and choose clear quality standards.

L. Hakvoort (✉)
Music Therapy Department, ArtEZ University of the Arts, Enschede, The Netherlands
e-mail: L.Hakvoort@artez.nl

U. Volpe (ed.), *Arts Therapies in Psychiatric Rehabilitation*,
https://doi.org/10.1007/978-3-030-76208-7_8

For most music therapists worldwide, collecting evidence-based information regarding MT also implies to translate the retrieved evidence to their own and their client's cultural context [13, 14]. An important realization is awareness of the cultural and ideological focus towards MT of the person executing the review. The review by Windle and Carr [15] is nicely colored by the humanistic/psychodynamic view on MT treatment from Great-Britain and Nordic countries, focusing on the client's well-being and facilitating growth through the musical therapeutic relation. Lately the awareness of culture-specific approaches in MT has been emphasized, especially when treating clients with mental health issues [16]. The World Federation for Music Therapy incorporates that in their definition of MT; "Research, practice, education, and clinical training in music therapy are based on professional standards according to cultural, social, and political contexts" [14]. So cultural awareness is extremely important when defining evidence-based MT and specific approaches in MT profession [13].

In a review, literature on culturally sensitive MT approach for populations struggling with mental health issues due to oppression have to be included. Recent new perspectives like "queer theory" could be helpful to move beyond rigid classifications, and oppose pathologizing people with multiple, intersecting marginalized identities, such as those who are disabled, ethnic minorities, etc. [17, 18]. New research should study whether pathologizing clients towards diagnostic criteria would be helpful for their improved functioning and the role of MT in this process. Harris [19] provides a qualitative description on how queering a therapeutic musical alliance can decrease power differences between the client and therapist. A review requires a music therapist to dive deep into new material, to understand the offered approach and link it to their client's cultural responsivity.

Another important aspect of reviewing MT evidence would be diving into the latest insights of its working mechanisms. Windle and Carr [15] emphasize the role of the therapist in MT for social well-being goals in mental health. Foubert et al. [20] stretch the emotional and therapeutic relatedness of clients with borderline personality disorder in MT treatment, as do Hannibal et al. [21]. Bensimon [22] formulates the specific musical attuned involvement and validation as well as musical witnessing as the most important relation-strengthening aspects of MT intervention. Although social and emotional functions of music and the therapeutic alliance are well-defined in most studies, the neurologic understanding of possible working mechanisms of the music itself are hardly explained. Interestingly, Leubner and Hinterberger [23] found in their systematic review of MT versus music-based interventions for depression, that the person who shaped the intervention was not really important. The music intervention itself showed significant positive changes in mood for people with depression. Understanding the neurologic mechanisms of music is essential when providing evidence-based MT in practice.

One of the more recent MT treatments and (acclaimed) evidence-based MT approach that has its main emphasis on the neurologic impact of music on the brain is the Neurologic music therapy (NMT, [24]). In the NMT, the role of the music as cue for neurologic therapeutic processes is eminent. Although developed for neurorehabilitation especially the cognitive treatment interventions of the NMT, like

Musical Attention Control Training (MACT, [25]), seem to meet the needs of clients with mental health issues. Clients with schizophrenia and psychosis often show deficits to focus or sustain attention, or have problems to select adequate information [26–28]. Improvement of attention could be correlated with better treatment outcomes [26]. A randomized controlled study with forensic psychiatric patients with psychotic features showed significant improvement in their sustained and selective attention after 6 one-hour MACT group interventions [29]. These outcomes copied the results of an unpublished study of MACT for a similar population by Roefs [30].

In the NMT, the neurologic mechanisms of how music can drive attention take precedence [31]. BRECVEMA[1]-mechanisms (music triggered neurologic mechanisms; [32]) activated during MACT are (1) brainstem reflex, generated by changes in music's volume, silence, shape, tonality, intervals, tempo; (2) musical entrainment, cued by steady pulse, clear measures, rhythmical patterns; and (3) musical expectancy, prompted by timing, tonality, shaping [32].

For patients with post-traumatic stress disorders (PTSD), trauma-informed music therapy interventions are developed [33]. One of the interventions recently investigated in two feasibility studies is the Short-term Music therapy Attention and Arousal Regulation Training (SMAART, [34]). This six-session-music-based-intervention, administered by accredited music therapists, shows promising results. The first study for incarcerated psychiatric patients with PTSD showed an improved selective and sustained attention, as well as reduced arousal symptoms [35]. A similar study with SMAART including day-treatment clients diagnosed with PTSD and substance use disorder, showed equal results regarding attention and arousal, but a larger drop-out rate [36]. In each of these studies, the assumed (neurologic) working mechanisms of the music is defined as core part of the MT intervention.

To ensure improved evidence-based MT treatment in the near future, MT interventions require a more explicit definition of the neurological mechanisms triggered by the music. If music therapeutic interventions should meet the most recent understanding of mental functioning of the clients, it is essential to formulate them culturally sensitive and focus on the music-neurologic mechanisms. This requires that music therapy interventions are formulated culture-sensitive, in detail, and the neurologic (working) mechanisms of the music are defined comprehensively [37, 38].

References

1. Coomans A. Moments in music therapy—a review of different concepts and connotations in music therapy. Musikther Umsch. 2018;39(4):337–53.
2. Wang S, Agius M. The use of music therapy in the treatment of mental illness and the enhancement of societal wellbeing. Psychiatr Danub. 2018;30(Suppl 7):595–600.

[1]BRECVEMA stands for Brainstem reflex, Rhythmical entrainment, Evaluative conditioning, Contagion, Visual imagery, Episodic memory, Musical expectancy, and Aesthetic Judgement (see [32]).

3. McCaffrey T. Evaluating music therapy in adult mental health services: tuning into service user perspectives. Nord J Music Ther. 2018;27(1):28–43.
4. Paul N, Lotter C, van Staden W. Patient reflections on individual music therapy for a major depressive disorder or acute phase schizophrenia spectrum disorder. J Music Ther. 2020;57(2):168–92.
5. Bibb J, Castle D, McFerran KS. Stakeholder input into the implementation of a new music therapy program in a mental health service. Ment Health Rev J. 2018;23(4):293–307. https://doi.org/10.1108/MHRJ-12-2017-0056.
6. Pedersen IN, Bonde LO, Hannibal NJ, Nielsen J, Aagaard J, Bertelsen LR, et al. Music therapy as treatment of negative symptoms for adult patients diagnosed with schizophrenia—study protocol for a randomized, controlled and blinded study. Medicines. 2019;6(2):46.
7. Silverman MJ. Music therapy for coping self-efficacy in an acute mental health setting: a randomized pilot study. Community Ment Health J. 2019a;55(4):615–23.
8. Volpe U, Gianoglio C, Autiero L, Marino ML, Facchini D, Mucci A, Galderisi S. Acute effects of music therapy in subjects with psychosis during inpatient treatment. Psychiatry. 2018;81(3):218–27.
9. Archambault K, Vaugon K, Deumié V, Brault M, Perez RM, Peyrin J, et al. MAP: a personalized receptive music therapy intervention to improve the affective well-being of youths hospitalized in a mental health unit. J Music Ther. 2019;56(4):381–402.
10. Hense C, Silverman MJ, McFerran KS. Using the healthy-unhealthy uses of music scale as a single-session music therapy intervention on an acute youth mental health inpatient unit. Music Ther Perspect. 2018;36(2):267–76.
11. Rosado A. Adolescents' experiences of music therapy in an inpatient crisis stabilization unit. Music Ther Perspect. 2019;37(2):133–40.
12. Quinn K. Heavy metal music and managing mental health: heavy metal therapy. Metal Music Stud. 2019;5(3):419–24.
13. Belgrave M, Kim S-A. Music therapy in a multicultural context: a handbook for music therapy students and professionals. London, UK: Jessica Kingsley Publisher; 2020.
14. WFMT (World Federation of Music Therapy). Definition of music therapy. 2011. https://www.wfmt.info//wp-content/uploads/2014/05/ENGLISH-NEW-What-is-music-therapy.pdf. Accessed 1 Feb 2021.
15. Windle E, Carr C. Music therapy in psychiatry. In: Volpe U, editor. Art therapies in psychiatric rehabilitation. London: Springer; 2021.
16. Abdulbaki H, Berger J. Using culture-specific music therapy to manage the therapy deficit of post-traumatic stress disorder and associated mental health conditions in Syrian refugee host environments. Approaches. 2020;12(2). ISSN: 2459-3338.
17. Bain C, Gumble M. Querying dialogues: a performative editorial on queering music therapy. Voices. 2019;19(3) https://doi.org/10.15845/voices.v19i3.2904.
18. Whitehead-Pleaux A. Queering music therapy: music therapy and LGBTQAI+ peoples. In: Hogan S, editor. Arts therapies and gender issues: international perspectives on research. New York, NY: Routledge; 2019. p. 22–36.
19. Harris B. Queer as a bell: music and the psychotherapeutic relationship. Voices. 2019;19(3) https://doi.org/10.15845/voices.v19i3.2674.
20. Foubert K, Sebreghts B, Sutton J, De Backer J. Musical encounters on the borderline. Patterns of mutuality in musical improvisations with borderline personality disorder. Arts Psychother. 2020;67 https://doi.org/10.1016/j.aip.2019.101599.
21. Hannibal N, Nygaard Pedersen I, Bonde L, Bertelsen L. A pilot study investigating research design feasibility using pre-post measures to test the effect of music therapy in psychiatry with people diagnosed with personality disorders. Voices. 2019;19(1) https://doi.org/10.15845/voices.v19i1.2731.
22. Bensimon M. Relational needs in music therapy with trauma victims: the perspective of music therapists. Nord J Music Ther. 2020;29(3):240–54.
23. Leubner D, Hinterberger T. Reviewing the effectiveness of music interventions in treating depression. Front Psychol. 2017;8:1109. https://doi.org/10.3389/fpsyg.2017.01109.

24. Thaut M, Hoemberg V, editors. Handbook of neurologic music therapy. Oxford, UK: University Press; 2014.
25. Thaut, M. H., & Gardiner, J. C. (2014). Musical attention control training. In: M.H. Thaut & V. Hoemberg (Eds.). Handbook of neurologic music therapy (pg. 257–269). Oxford, UK: University Press.
26. Cornet LJM, Van der Laan PH, Nijman HLI, Tollenaar N, De Kogel CH. Neurobiological factors as predictors of prisoners'. Response to a cognitive skills training. J Crim Just. 2015;43:122–32. https://doi.org/10.1016/j.jcrimjus.2015.02.003.
27. Kavanagh L, Rowe D, Hersch J, Barnett KJ, Reznik R. Neurocognitive deficits and psychiatric disorders in a NSW prison population. Int J Law Psychiatry. 2010;33:20–6. https://doi.org/10.1016/j.ijlp.2009.10.004.
28. Meyer G, Spray A, Fairlie J, Uomini N. Inferring common cognitive mechanisms from brain blood-flow lateralisation data: a new methodology for fTCD analysis. Front Psychol. 2014;5:552. https://doi.org/10.3389/fpsyg.2014.00552.
29. Van Alphen R, Stams GJ, Hakvoort L. Musical attention control training for psychotic psychiatric patients: an experimental pilot study in a forensic psychiatric hospital. Front Neurosci. 2019;13:570.
30. Roefs G. Neurologische muziektherapie en schizofrenie [Neurologic music therapy and schizophrenia]. 2015. https://kenvak.nl/wp-content/uploads/2015/04/2015-06-26-Gerben-Roefs-Eindpresentatie-Neurologische-Muziektherapie-bij-Schizofrenie.pdf. Accessed 1 Feb 2021.
31. Thaut M, Hodges DA. The Oxford handbook of music and the brain. Oxford, UK: University Press; 2019.
32. Juslin PN. Musical emotions explained: unlocking the secrets of musical affect. Oxford, UK: University Press; 2019.
33. Behrens GA. Challenges, benefits, and trends from a neurobiological approach to music therapy. Music Ther Today. 2019;15(1):13–20. https://issuu.com/presidentwfmt/docs/mt_today._2019. Accessed 1 Feb 2021.
34. Macfarlane C. Development of the SMAART protocol for adult male prisoners with PTSD. Music Ther Today. 2019;15(1):21–32. https://issuu.com/presidentwfmt/docs/mt_today._2019. Accessed 1 Feb 2021.
35. Macfarlane C, Masthoff E, Hakvoort L. Short-term music therapy attention and arousal regulation treatment (SMAART) for prisoners with posttraumatic stress disorder: a feasibility study. J Forensic Psychol Res Pract. 2019;19(5):376–92.
36. Hakvoort L, de Jong S, van de Ree M, Kok T, Macfarlane C, de Haan H. Short-term music therapy for patients with substance use and PTSD: a pilot study for hyperarousal and attention. J Music Ther. 2020;57(3):353–78.
37. Hakvoort L, Tönjes, D. Music-mechanisms at the core of music therapy: towards a format for micro-description of music therapy interventions (in review).
38. Hakvoort L, Van der Eng C. Micro-interventies voor de vaktherapeutische beroepen [Micro-intervention for arts therapies]. Tijdschrift voor Vaktherapie. 2020;16(1):14–21.

Recurring Sound Aspects in Group Work with Psychiatric Patients

9

Diana Facchini and Gianluca Catuogno

In Italy, music therapy (MT) with psychiatric patients reflects a wide variety of experiences. We generally agree with ongoing international studies and research, thoroughly reviewed by Carr and Windle, reporting positive effects of MT on many neuropsychiatric disorders, including affective and psychotic syndromes [1, 2].

The *Istituto formazione di musicoterapia* (Isfom; [3]) is a historical educational reality in Italy, that has encouraged and supported MT activities for many years, in close connection with psychiatric territorial structures. The results of such activity showed short- or medium-term benefits compared to the global health state, mental health state, functioning and quality of life of patients with psychiatric disorders [4]. In group settings, it is clear that MT is considered as a mean to increase cohesion, acceptance, and interpersonal relationships and is considered as an additional psychosocial treatment for psychosis, more effective than mere pharmacological therapy alone [4, 5].

The basic principle that regulates MT interventions in psychiatry is linked to the exploration of the self, the mobilization of affects, the development of the creative and cognitive parts, and the release of blocked energy nuclei. MT represents an encounter between people, made of emotions and memories that are generated in a real and symbolic space (MT setting), according to the definition that Winnicott gives of the traditional psychoanalytic situation [6], which evokes propitiatory rites

D. Facchini (✉)
"ISFOM—Istituto Formazione Musicoterapia", Naples, Italy

University "L. Vanvitelli", Naples, Italy
e-mail: info@isfom.it

G. Catuogno
"ISFOM—Istituto Formazione Musicoterapia", Naples, Italy

"Pediatric Pain Service and Palliative Care" of A.O.R.N. Santobono-Pausilipon, Naples, Italy
e-mail: gianluca@capri.it

U. Volpe (ed.), *Arts Therapies in Psychiatric Rehabilitation*,
https://doi.org/10.1007/978-3-030-76208-7_9

of catharsis and healing. The intersubjective relationship between *operator* and *client* is based on empathy. This is the unique emotional attunement and goes beyond the specific action of music [7].

In line with the plurality of international music therapy models, the Isfom methodology is inspired by Benenzon's psychodynamic approach with additions to the humanistic and cognitive behavioral methodologies of Anglo-Saxon schools [4, 8]; it also makes particular reference to ethnomusicological aspects due to its strong epistemological component.

A recent research work carried out in collaboration with the Department of Mental Health of University "L. Vanvitelli" (Naples, Italy), at the local emergency psychiatric ward, allowed to quantitatively assess the results of MT provision in emergency settings and to observe recurring elements of such activity, reporting overall favorable results in the short term for patients with severe mental illnesses. In more detail, a repeated analysis of the variance measurements revealed that the patients undergoing music therapy treatment showed a statistically significant reduction in the Brief Psychiatric Rating Scale (BPRS) and Clinical Global Impression (CGI) scores, compared to the control group. Furthermore, after the observation period, the "anxiety/depression" factor of BPRS and the Hospital Anxiety Depression Scale (HADS) scores for affective symptoms decreased significantly [9].

In this work, as in similar protocols carried out by Isfom along the years, a specific instrumentation is needed. The Orff instruments and those from popular tradition are added to the piano, with specific reference to the four basic natural elements, to the female vs. male dimension, and to evocation of archetypal symbols [10]. This setting is crucial to support "images" and "musical conduct" [11] that regularly emerge within this MT approach. The sounds generated tend to repeat themselves in a kaleidoscopic form, favoring recurring structures and loops regarding rhythms, intervals, and melodies. The MT session usually starts with a direct approach to the instruments that Lecourt defines as *sound brouillage* [12], the initial moment of experimentation, generally long in duration and sometimes chaotic; in our case, this activity is linked to a few exploratory instants, due to the willingness to come into sound contact early [13].

Within our approach, rhythm emerges as a *phenomenon of motor induction*, linked to a desire for pleasure and contentment [14]. Only from the rhythmic experimentation the other phases develop, always linked to melody, vocality, and sound dramatization. In some cases, rhythmic production remains the aggregating element of communication.

The introspective vocality, which does not generally appear in an initial phase of work, immediately emerges in the form of songs, vocalizations, screams, and onomatopoeias. Patients tend to spontaneously let emerge their emotions and tell personal stories in music. The work on improvised singing is outlined by the presence of known songs and, subsequently, with a free repertoire. Songs, such as the traditional *tammurriata*, are a constant in the production of each group, linked to the popular cultural identity (according to the "ISO principle"; [15]) and to a rhythmic-melodic material perceived as familiar and reassuring. At the same time, they are linked to the need to externalize inner thoughts, deep feelings, and emotionally loaded themes such as addiction, sexuality-related issues, anger feelings, or gender contrasts. Based on the 4/4 "slogan" rhythm, recurring in most musical cultures and linked to movements of walking/swinging, such musical production is repleted with instinct, that unites automatic movements with biological rhythms. These rhythms, as they are expressed within a collective action, put in place a natural synchronization for the group members and create a strong emotional resonance. Satisfaction is reinforced in the socialization of rhythmic conduct. This mechanism may be often seen as a sort of *compulsion to repeat* musical patterns [16] and pushes the group to maintain vitality and narcissistic desire in the relationship. Later on, usually the group progresses and stabilizes.

Among the framed drums (privileged to represent figures, scenes, characters), the *ocean drum* emerges, a musical instrument evocative of the amniotic fluid (connected to the dimension of motherhood, letting feel the improviser as being a child), which allows deep emotions facilitated by music therapists.

Smeijsters [17] has written extensively on the theme of the affinity between musical processes and expressive properties, on the one hand, and on the processes of human life and pathological characteristics, on the other, highlighting analogies between pathological problems and behavioral patterns. The emotional sound response, expressed by the patients, represents their very transformational pathway. All musical elements are retained, within this conceptual framework, as specific symbolic equivalents of the non-musical elements of human behavior and interaction. Smeijsters also coined the dual concept of "musical pathological processes" and "musical therapeutic processes" [17]. The author underlines how the overall experience and knowledge of these analogies makes it possible to decide to what extent MT is a more or less appropriate treatment and indicates the affinities between analogy, diagnosis, indications and objectives, procedures and techniques of treatment.

In our experience with psychiatric patients, particularly those with acute syndromes, music therapy plays a special role in enhancing creativity and well-being, facilitating emotional sharing, favoring the transformation of painful perceptions, helping in anxiety containment, listening one to another, and uplifting the sense of belonging to the group and personal identity.

References

1. Silverman MJ. The influence of music on the symptoms of psychosis: a meta-analysis. J Music Ther. 2003;40(1):27–40.
2. Lu SF, Lo CH, Sung HC, Hsieh TC, Yu SC, Chang SC. Effects of group music intervention on psychiatric symptoms and depression inpatient with schizophrenia. Complement Ther Med. 2013;21(6):682–8.
3. Di Franco G. La scuola napoletana – Un modello per la formazione. Napoli: Isfom; 2002.
4. Di Franco G. Le voci dell'emozione. Roma: Ismez; 2001.
5. Mössler K, Chen X, Heldal TO, Gold C. Music therapy for people with schizophrenia and schizophrenia-like disorders. Cochrane Database Syst Rev. 2011;(12):CD004025.

6. Winnicott D. Through pediatrics to psychoanalysis: collected papers. London: Taylor & Francis; 1992.
7. Stern DN. The present moment in psychotherapy and everyday life. Ney Work/London: Norton; 2004.
8. Benenzon RO, De Ganza VH, Wagner G. La nuova musicoterapia. Roma: Phoenix; 1997.
9. Volpe U, Gianoglio C, Autiero L, Marino ML, Facchini D, Mucci A, Galderisi S. Acute effects of music therapy in subjects with psychosis during inpatient treatment. Psychiatry. 2018;81(3):218–27.
10. Jung CG. Gli archetipi dell'inconscio collettivo. Milano: Bollati Boringhieri; 1977.
11. Delalande F. Le condotte musicali/Les conduites musicales. Bologna: Clueb; 1986.
12. Lecourt E. Analisi di gruppo e musicoterapia. Assisi: Cittadella; 1996.
13. Bion WR. Analisi degli schizofrenici e metodo psicoanalitico. Roma: Armando; 2009.
14. Cano C. Il valore simbolico e il potere trasformativo della musica nel mito. In: Assenza C, Passannanti B, editors. Musica, storia, Cultura ed Educazione. Milano: Franco Angeli; 2001.
15. Benenzon RO. Etica del non verbale. Roma: Borla; 2020.
16. Fraisse P. Psicologia del ritmo. Roma: Armando; 1979.
17. Smeijsters, H. Developing concepts for a general theory of music therapy. Music as representation, replica, semi-rapresentation, symbol, metaphor, semisymbol, isomorphé, and analogy. 4° European music therapy conference, Leuwen. 1998.

10 Introducing Mechanisms of Music Therapy for People with Dementia: A Commentary to Music Therapy Chapter by Carr and Windle

Paolo Pizziolo

10.1 Commentary

Having practised as a music therapist for 19 years with people living with dementia and mental health pathologies, and as a PhD candidate in music therapy at Anglia Ruskin University, I found that Windle and Carr's essay is a valuable introduction to music therapy in mental health. The authors' concise and effective presentation of music therapy in mental health research and practice leads to considerations regarding the internal mechanisms of the music therapy process in the practice of music therapy and music therapy research.

Windle and Carr presented reviews and studies of music therapy related to mental health across a broad range of clinical areas [schizophrenia and psychosis, depression and anxiety, dementia, post-traumatic stress disorder (PTSD) and refugees, addiction and substance misuse, perinatal mental health, forensic psychiatry, child and adolescent mental health, and mixed-diagnosis groups]. The reviews of RCTs in many of these areas seem to indicate that investigating the internal mechanisms of music therapy might become a pre-eminent topic in a variety of Music Therapy (MT) research areas, especially in the mental health field where it is crucial to understand exactly how music therapy can impact emotion regulation [1–3].

In the research literature, a "mechanism" generally indicates identified procedures which can explain the phenomena observed [4]. In the field of music psychology, the concept of an underlying mechanism refers to a functional description of what the mind does when music evokes a certain type of emotion [5]. Juslin and colleagues explained musical emotions as being triggered by different types of information in musical events that activated a set of eight underlying mechanisms defined by the acronym BRECVMA [6], which stands for *Brain stem reflex*,

P. Pizziolo (✉)
Anglia Ruskin University, Cambridge Institute for Music Therapy Research, Cambridge, UK

U. Volpe (ed.), *Arts Therapies in Psychiatric Rehabilitation*,
https://doi.org/10.1007/978-3-030-76208-7_10

Rhythmic entrainment, *Evaluative conditioning*, *Contagion*, *Visual imagery*, *Episodic memory*, *Musical expectancy*, and *Aesthetic judgment*.

In music therapy research, the term mechanism is used to describe the physical and/or psychological effects of music therapy [1, 5, 7–9]. Fachner [10, 11] highlighted that mechanisms involved in music therapy practice can be explained through the use of neuroscientific methods such as electroencephalogram (EEG) and neuroimaging.

In the philosophy of science [12], a mechanism is described as a framework concept which includes a variety of models. Most of the models work by describing how the "parts, causal interactions, and organization features" [12] of phenomena are related to each other in producing the phenomena. From this perspective, a mechanism should be studied by deconstructing it into its components. This framework concept of mechanisms seems to be the most useful for studying the underlying mechanism in music therapy because it allows the relationship between the various mechanism components and types of evidence to be taken into account.

The evidence-based music therapy approach favours methodologies of difference-making (such as randomized clinical trials and meta-analyses). The Cochrane 2011 and 2017 [13, 14] reviews of MT and Dementia RCTs highlighted their limitations. In the 2011 review, the authors did not consider it possible to determine whether to advise MT or not and in the 2017 review, the evidence was deemed to be scarce. In general, it was noted that there was a need for more robust RCT studies (for example, the statistical reporting of the studies' outcomes was considered poor [13]). The 2017 Cochrane Review [14] found low-quality evidence that music-based therapeutic interventions may have little or no effect on emotional well-being and quality of life, overall behaviour problems and cognition and found moderate-quality evidence that they reduce depressive symptoms. Dissatisfaction was also expressed regarding the quality of reporting as it was lacking detailed information about the intervention. This was in line with previous reviews [6, 7, 13, 14] which also highlighted the importance of describing the music therapy process and the underlying mechanisms of music therapy.

Given the nature of MT, evidence is of various types and on more than one level, and it is probable that the two different knowledge-related approaches, knowing that A is a cause of B and knowing how A causes B, need to be used in an integrated way to design RCTs which should incorporate mixed methods to better identify the outcomes to be measured. To further integrate the two different types of knowledge, the idea introduced by Schall [15] of investigating and measuring what happens within a single session using a time series as well as pre-post measures of the session set under study might be further developed.

Windle and Carr outline that MT therapy outcomes in mental health therapies, including for dementia, should not be limited to considerations regarding symptomatic relief. The authors correctly highlight that in assessing music therapy outcomes, it is crucial to consider multiple types of evidence, particularly the therapeutic relationship and micro-level events during the therapeutic process, and identify what works best. This way of identifying the underlying mechanisms of MT, especially in music therapy for Persons with Dementia (PWD), is in line with the framework concept of mechanisms introduced in philosophy of science [12] and responds to an essential need in research on music therapy with PWD [16–18].

Music therapy with PWD is primarily aimed at reducing Behavioural and Psychological Symptoms of Dementia (BPSD), at maintaining their cognitive functions and improving their quality of life [19]. A recent study [20] used a mixed methods approach to investigate mechanisms of BPSD reduction in group music therapy with PWD and included music therapy techniques (according to Bruscia's [21] taxonomy), environmental conditions and relationships as Moments of BPSD Reduction (MBR) mechanism components. The study identified a two-phase mechanism for MBRs, where the *Rhythmic Grounding*, *Pacing*, and *Making Spaces* techniques worked together with specific features of the clinical environment to predispose conditions for MBRs (first phase). Then other mechanism components regarding the group's therapeutic relationships, atmosphere and environment; extra-musical phenomena; the need for music therapist flexibility; and music therapy ingredients and techniques (such as *Calming*, *Pacing*, and *Rhythmic Grounding* and *Introducing Change*) all functioned to achieve MBRs (second phase). The *Rhythmic Grounding* technique was a constant component of MBRs in all phases and conditions.

This mixed methods study is one of the first of the many more that will be needed to glean additional insights into how music therapy outcomes are achieved in mental health and dementia.

References

1. Legge AW. On the neural mechanisms of music therapy in mental health care: literature review and clinical implications. MTPERS. 2015;33:128–41. https://doi.org/10.1093/mtp/miv025.
2. Mastnak W. Perinatal music therapy and antenatal music classes: principles, mechanisms, and benefits. J Perinat Educ. 2016;25:184–92. https://doi.org/10.1891/1058-1243.25.3.184.
3. Juslin PN, Harmat L, Eerola T. What makes music emotionally significant? Exploring the underlying mechanisms. Psychol Music. 2014;42:599–623. https://doi.org/10.1177/0305735613484548.
4. Robson C. Real world research: a resource for users of social research methods in applied settings. Chichester, West Sussex: Wiley; 2011.
5. Hallam S, Cross I, Thaut M. The Oxford handbook of music psychology. Oxford: University Press, Incorporated; 2018.
6. Juslin PN, Västfjäll D. Emotional responses to music: the need to consider underlying mechanisms. Behav Brain Sci. 2008;31:559–75. https://doi.org/10.1017/S0140525X08005293.
7. Fang R, Ye S, Huangfu J, Calimag DP. Music therapy is a potential intervention for cognition of Alzheimer's disease: a mini-review. Transl Neurodegener. 2017;6 https://doi.org/10.1186/s40035-017-0073-9.
8. Clements-Cortes A, Bartel L. Are we doing more than we know? Possible mechanisms of response to music therapy. Front Med. 2018;5 https://doi.org/10.3389/fmed.2018.00255.
9. Thaut MH, McIntosh GC, Hoemberg V. Neurobiological foundations of neurologic music therapy: rhythmic entrainment and the motor system. Front Psychol. 2015;5 https://doi.org/10.3389/fpsyg.2014.01185.
10. Fachner J. The future of music therapy and neuroscience. In: Di Leo C, editor. Envisioning the future of music therapy. Philadelphia, PA: Temple University; 2016. p. 139–48.

11. Fachner J, Gold C, Erkkilä J. Music therapy modulates fronto-temporal activity in rest-EEG in depressed clients. Brain Topogr. 2013;26:338–54. https://doi.org/10.1007/s10548-012-0254-x.
12. Craver C, Tabery J. Mechanisms in science. In: Zalta EN, editor. The Stanford encyclopedia of philosophy, summer 2019. Stanford: Metaphysics Research Lab, Stanford University; 2019. https://plato.stanford.edu/archives/sum2019/entries/science-mechanisms/. Accessed 3 Sept 2020.
13. Vink AC, Bruinsma MS, Scholten RJ. Music therapy for people with dementia. Cochrane Database Syst Rev. 2011;(3) https://doi.org/10.1002/14651858.CD003477.pub2.
14. van der Steen JT, van Soest-Poortvliet MC, van der Wouden JC, Bruinsma MS, Scholten RJ, Vink AC. Music-based therapeutic interventions for people with dementia. In: The Cochrane Collaboration, editor. Cochrane database of systematic reviews. Chichester, UK: John Wiley & Sons, Ltd; 2017. https://doi.org/10.1002/14651858.CD003477.pub3.
15. Schall A, Haberstroh J, Pantel J. Time series analysis of individual music therapy in dementia: effects on communication behavior and emotional well-being. GeroPsych. 2015;28:113–22. https://doi.org/10.1024/1662-9647/a000123.
16. McDermott O, Crellin N, Ridder HM, Orrell M. Music therapy in dementia: a narrative synthesis systematic review. Int J Geriatr Psychiatry. 2012; https://doi.org/10.1002/gps.3895.
17. Vasionytė I, Madison G. Musical intervention for patients with dementia: a meta-analysis. J Clin Nurs. 2013;22:1203–16. https://doi.org/10.1111/jocn.12166.
18. Gold C, Eickholt J, Assmus J, Stige B, Wake JD, Baker FA, Tamplin J, Clark I, Lee Y-EC, Jacobsen SL, Ridder HMO, Kreutz G, Muthesius D, Wosch T, Ceccato E, Raglio A, Ruggeri M, Vink A, Zuidema S, Odell-Miller H, Orrell M, Schneider J, Kubiak C, Romeo R, Geretsegger M. Music Interventions for Dementia and Depression in ELderly care (MIDDEL): protocol and statistical analysis plan for a multinational cluster-randomised trial. BMJ Open. 2019;9:e023436. https://doi.org/10.1136/bmjopen-2018-023436.
19. Hsu MH, Flowerdew R, Parker M, Fachner J, Odell-Miller H. Individual music therapy for managing neuropsychiatric symptoms for people with dementia and their carers: a cluster randomised controlled feasibility study. BMC Geriatr. 2015;15:84. https://doi.org/10.1186/s12877-015-0082-4.
20. Pizziolo P. Investigating the role of music therapy in the reduction of behavioural and psychological symptoms for people with dementia. Doctoral dissertation, Anglia Ruskin University. 2019. https://arro.anglia.ac.uk/id/eprint/706018/. Accessed 4 Nov 2020.
21. Bruscia KE. Improvisational models of music therapy. Springfield, IL: C.C. Thomas; 1987.

Part III

Dance Movement Therapy

Integration in Motion: Dance Movement Therapy

11

Hilda Wengrower and Talia Bendel-Rozow

11.1 Introduction

Dance movement therapy (DMT) is a professional approach to enhance the psycho-physical, social, emotional, and cognitive integration of the person in order to advance their health and well-being [1]. Dance movement therapy is based on the confluence of knowledge stemming from the practice and lived experience of dance and the concepts and models psychology provided in its different branches. In the last decades, neuroscience and cognitive science have contributed to strengthening the validity of DMT's earliest fundamental principles.

11.1.1 History of Dance Movement Therapy

For centuries, dance has been used in rituals aimed at community cohesion and averting the bad spirits assumed to be behind sickness. The creation of the world was described as a dance of god (i.e., Siva Nataraja) in India. Roman poet Lucian (second century CE) considered dance to be the richest offering of the Muses to humankind and a mirror of universal harmony [2].

Rituals praying to nature's forces for rain, group empowerment before going to hunt or to war, celebration of good harvests, and more events were mostly danced. According to the ancient concepts of body–mind–spirit unity, shamans and witch healers danced to cure various afflictions—until the Cartesian dualism separating mind from body spread through Western culture [3]. Even though culture considered the body impure, dance remained an essential part of rural life in celebrations,

H. Wengrower (✉)
School for Society and Arts, Ono Academic College, Kiryat Ono, Israel
e-mail: mshilda@mail.huji.ac.il

T. Bendel-Rozow
Herzliya, Israel

U. Volpe (ed.), *Arts Therapies in Psychiatric Rehabilitation*,
https://doi.org/10.1007/978-3-030-76208-7_11

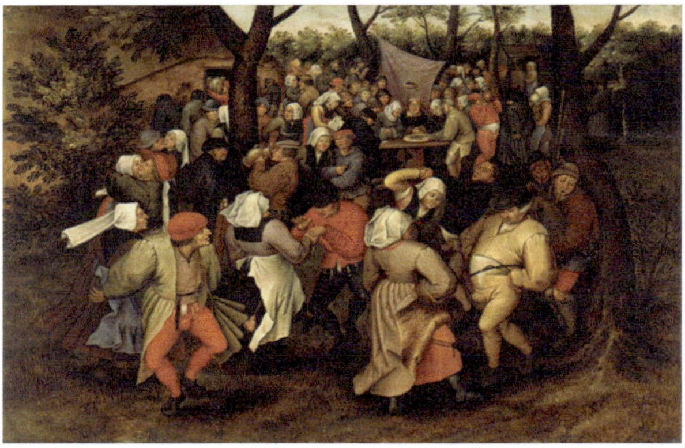

Fig. 11.1 Peasant wedding dance (P. Bruegel II, 1607). (This work has been released into the public domain by Walters Art Museum)

as Pieter Brueghel's II painting, *Peasant dance* (Fig. 11.1), clearly depicts. Even in Western countries, residuals of rural healing dances were practiced until the first part of the twentieth century. One such case in Southern Italy is *tarantism*, a disease thought to be caused by the bite of the tarantula spider, characterized by a variety of psychosomatic symptoms (including pains, breathlessness, palpitations, emotional lability, and unusual sexual urges). Tarantism traditionally was cured with long sessions (sometimes until the subject's exhaustion) of rhythmic dance to the doleful sound of the *tarantella* [4].

As a modern profession, DMT developed due to the confluence of several factors that, as in any complex process, interact and overlap. One of the first contributions to the current form of DMT arose from the evolution of classical ballet into modern dance. The late nineteenth and early twentieth centuries saw a break from former aesthetic values and structures: personal expression, noncodified movements and gestures, and releasing body and clothing were dominating the scene [5]. Mary Wigman, a revolutionary in dance, saw in this art a path to self-knowledge and personal development. She included expression of the person's dark aspects, as in her dance, "The Witch" [6].

Another founding contribution to the modern conceptualization of DMT is that of Rudolf Laban's philosophy and his vision about dance and movement. Laban's approach had an influence of great magnitude on acting, dancing, and education through the arts. Around the turn of the twentieth century (beginning of the modernist era in the arts), there was hope for an absolute and scientific language to access reality. At the same time, under the burgeoning psychoanalysis and expressionism, the arts searched for ways to uncover the artists' subjectivity. One result of this polarity was that rationality and mental operations were attributed to the mind, whereas intuitions, emotions, and imagination were ascribed to the body [7]. Laban clearly opposed this dichotomy. He strived to integrate the rational and the irrational in the human being. Neglecting the latter would drive a person to lose control of the personal life and fall into a state of insecurity that is hard to remedy.

The vital impulses are mixed; they appear in physical and mental activities. Laban urged his readers and followers to be aware of their emotions and thoughts

[8, 9]. He saw in movement a testimony to life's bipolarity: In daily tasks, it is possible to see components of the dream world. Laban probably was aware of Freud's writings about art when he presented it as the sublimation and condensation of irrational impulses. A dance in which an individual or a group pursue authentic expression sets a basis for communion with nature, like contemplation and generates inner peace.

Also of great relevance to the development of DMT is the contribution of the psychoanalytic tradition; the notion of the unconscious had a great impact on psychiatry and on art. "The technique of free-association of words that Freud used in treating his patients is based on the notion that spontaneous expression allows unconscious aspects to appear, decreasing their repressive control" ([10], pp. 15–16). This technique entered the dance world through improvisation, probably as a transformation of *automatism*, a way of work surrealist artists used to create art. They relegated conscious awareness to retrieve material from the unconscious as part of the creative process. Psychoanalysts' analyses of art pieces, as well as their writings on art and the creative process, also may have influenced DMT's birth and expansion [10].

Nonverbal expression and communication long have been considered of high interest for both psychology and psychiatry. In *The Expression of the Emotions in Man and the Animals*, Darwin [11] scrutinized the geneses and functions of facial and bodily expression. Thus, he contributed to associating and diagnosing these expressions to mental illness. About a century after Darwin, Martha Davis established that movement reflects intrapsychic, interpersonal, and cultural patterns [12]. These are only a few examples of research inquiring into the meaning of nonverbal expression, which is one of the pillars of DMT.

From a purely historical perspective, the DMT timeline surely set a major mark throughout the first half of the twentieth century, with the need to provide psychiatric help for WWII veterans. This assistance was critical for the treatment and rehabilitation of thousands of former soldiers to overcome their traumas, live with their families, and return to civilian employment. Group work and innovative methods and therapies provided the solution—and DMT was one of those modalities [12].

To conclude the historical background of DMT, a place of honor should be kept for Marian Chace (1896–1970), one of the pioneers of DMT development in mental health settings. Still now, her perspective inspires and serves the work of dance movement therapists around the world, in mental health and with people of various ages and dissimilar needs. Her disciples, some of whom collaborated with her to found the American Dance Therapy Association, disseminated her teachings outside the United States. Following, aspects of Chace's life and work are presented with some detail. However, probably other persons (mostly women) also began a chain of DMT development in their own countries [13].

After dancing with the Denishawn company, Chace taught children and adolescents in a variety of settings. In her classes, she also met people who did not intend to have a career in dance. She became interested in their processes, shifting her focus from the technique to the person. In 1942, Chace was invited to work at the St. Elizabeth Psychiatric Hospital; 7 years later, she held there a full-time position as dance therapist, using dance for communication. In parallel, she studied psychodrama, took courses at the Washington School of Psychiatry directed by Frieda Fromm-Reichmann, and participated in the hospital's academic life. Chace practiced dance therapy for 20 years at St. Elizabeth Hospital and at Chestnut Lodge and taught briefly at the Rubin Academy of Music in Jerusalem and in Tel Aviv.

Chace maintained that dance must be ingrained in the therapist in order to use it for therapy. Her embodied knowledge as a dancer was the root from which she developed and systematized her work. Sharon Chaiklin [14] wrote about Chace's talent to observe nonverbal expression and to react to it in what later was called *empathic reflection* [15], giving the experience of being accepted and understood. Decades after Chace passed away, laboratory research reported on the positive influence on children in the autism spectrum when their gestures and movements were imitated by an adult [16]. Together with studies on mirror neurons [17], these findings provided research-based evidence supporting the theories and practices Chace had established (Box 11.1).

Box 11.1 Basic principles of Marian Chace's DMT [14]

- Tensions and distortions of the body reflect traumatic experience
- Readiness for change ("only when the [client] is ready for it will it become meaningful to him and effect a change in his body image")
- Movement symbolizes the unconscious (by reflecting and building on the movement offered, the patient could begin to claim the expression as his or her own and explore new possibilities)
- Integration of verbal and nonverbal communication ("flowing one into the other")
- Kinesthetic empathy
- Behavioral framework

Today, DMT constitutes an interdisciplinary profession with standardized training that, in most countries, is taught at the master's level. Although there are different professional associations around the globe, all study programs share a definite perspective related to movement and dance in a psychotherapeutic framework.

Implementation of DMT in psychiatric rehabilitation has followed diverse pathways throughout the world. Although most members of European and Asian DMT associations work in psychiatric settings, univocal information about worldwide DMT program implementation in psychiatric rehabilitation units is still difficult to find. In some countries, dance movement therapists are independent freelance employees, whereas in Australasia (Australia, New Zealand, and the Asian-Pacific region), a few work in rehabilitation. In other countries, such as Israel, DMT is implemented in both inpatient and outpatient psychiatric settings. The work in community-based rehabilitation settings is slowly growing following mental health policy legislation in 2015. The fundamental theoretical principles of DMT are presented briefly in the following section.

11.1.2 Fundamental Principles and Techniques

11.1.2.1 The Human Being Is Embodied

The French psychoanalyst Anzieu [18] stated that between 1950 and 1975 the body was absent from the discourse of different schools of psychotherapy as well as the realization of its being an essential aspect of human reality. The body's interconnection with the psyche, its liveliness, its dynamism in terms of the experience of emotions, interpersonal attractions, and rejections, wasn't recognized as such. Dance movement therapy brings to the fore the body—not the one observed and dissected by pathologists, but the lived, felt body.

Caldwell [19] recently stated that "being a body" implies humans are a polyphonic process of psycho-physiological functions, such as breathing, digesting, moving, feeling, and thinking. In this sense, the body is not something we "have" but rather "an experience we are." This is a sharp utterance within the psychiatric rehabilitation field, given that one of its aims is to further and maintain clients' achievements of being in their bodies, as well as to continue overcoming their dissociation and to help them experience the bodies that they are.

Winnicott [20] explored the human psyche-soma development within the context of relationship. He concluded that, in the course of psychosomatic integration, a process of reciprocal influences occur. According to his perspective, children delight in their progress in body functioning, which supports their ego development. This consequently "reinforces body functioning (influences muscle tone, coordination, adaptation to temperature change, etc.)" (p. 514). Because DMT is rooted in dance, it recognizes this reciprocity. This is one reason authors consider DMT to be a holistic psychotherapeutic modality [21, 22].

Seminal contributions from neuroscience long clarified that emotions "happen" first at the body level and then are transmitted to the brain by proprioceptive and interoceptive inputs [23]. Since the first stages of life, human beings know their environment, themselves, and others through nonsymbolic somatic experiences. Later, despite mastering the verbal realm, the implicit nonverbal knowledge never stops being active [24].

Fuchs and Koch [25] developed this idea further. They described their proposed construct of *embodied affectivity* as an embodied-relational affectivity in which the body is touched, moved, and affected by others' expressions. Within this model, the kinetics and intensity of emotions are perceived through kinesthetic sensations and interoceptive and proprioceptive feedback. Affects are not enclosed in the individual's mind; they are felt in the body. In turn, affects also are influenced in a relational intersomatic process. From a developmental perspective, the early care babies receive forms the basis for the implicit knowledge they have about themselves, their caretakers, and the environment. Therefore, borrowing an expression from Freud, we can state that the sense of self is a bodily sense achieved in the relation of the baby and its caretaker.

From a cognitive perspective, the enactive or embodied cognitive approaches sustain an integrative vision that overcomes the body–mind dualism by elaborating that self-organized processes that intersect brain, body, and environment set up cognition [26, 27]. To further overcome a dichotomic approach, one should consider that, rather than being a barrier to thinking, emotions are the basis for mental activities. Thus, DMT may be conceptualized as an enactive and embodied approach to therapy. It integrates emotion, perception, action, and cognition and operates on the patient's movement-pattern repertoire at a conscious and intersubjective level [28].

11.1.2.2 Body Awareness

A key concept of DMT that relates closely to embodiment is *body awareness*. This notion refers to "a subjective, phenomenological aspect of proprioception and interoception that enters consciousness and is modifiable by mental processes, including attention, interpretation, appraisal, beliefs, memories, conditioning, attitudes and affect" ([29], p. 1). Researchers have described the links between body awareness, emotion, and brain activity and considered the association between proprioception, interoception, and body awareness crucial for emotional regulation [30] and sense of self [31, 32]. Critchley et al. [33] stated that personal variation in the intensity of emotional states relates to differences in experiencing internal bodily reactions. Body awareness had been considered detrimental for patients prone to anxiety; however, there are reports of its favorable contribution for psychological adjustment [34].

Classically, DMT has been oriented to proprioception. Some years ago, Hindi [35] called on colleagues to integrate attention to enteroperception in their work with patients. Other authors more recently claimed that schizophrenia patients have low perceptivity to their inner physical signals. They suggested that "besides a feeble body ownership and an hyper/hypo-trophic sense of agency, the basic experience of the self, as a body self, in schizophrenia is also characterized by damaged interoceptive accuracy" ([36], p. 7).

11.1.2.3 Lived Meanings of Gesture, Posture, and Self-Knowledge

One corollary of the latter statement is that body and movement/dance are media of intra- and interpersonal communication; they carry implicit knowledge and procedural memory [10]. One work mode in DMT is encouraging patients to witness their emotions, physical sensations, associations, and images; move them; and then reflect on the experience with the therapist and/or the group and make connections with other aspects of their lives.

Dance movement therapy has several systems of movement observation that, together with the patient's self-report and anamnesis, guide the therapists in the dyadic interaction and allow them to produce profiles of the individual, assess the treatment process, and establish therapeutic goals. Gesture, posture, body attitude, and other body-movement features are observed, depicted, and assessed. As discussed earlier, Laban created one of the most-used systems of movement observation. Box 11.2 summarizes the basic aspects observed in Laban's system [37]. The Kestenberg Movement Profile added other components and integrated psychoanalysis into the interpretation of the observation. For a more in-depth discussion, see Loman and Sossin [38] and Sossin [39].

Box 11.2 Basic Aspects of Movement and Posture Observed in Movement Analysis Systems

- Use of body parts, alignment, movement of limbs/body center
- Use of personal space and of space in the room
- Mover's attitude to temporal components of movement: sudden/sustained
- Mover's attitude to strength: strong/light
- Mover's attitude to space: direct/indirect
- Bound/free flow of movement

Feniger-Schaal et al. [40] recently conducted a study on interpersonal interaction through play and movement by using the "mirror game" (i.e., the well-known game in which a participant imitates the movement and gestures of the other) as a source of information on the individual's attachment style. Because the mirror game is fundamentally an "interpersonal meeting," Feniger-Schaal et al. assumed that participants would play based on their procedural knowledge about a dyadic interaction and the many ways to carry out this exchange (such as synchronization, self-regulation, and use of interpersonal space). The researchers hypothesized that participants' performance of the game would reveal their attachment style—as indeed the study demonstrated. In a way, the experiment resembled part of a DMT session with people in psychiatric rehabilitation settings. The inquiry revealed that people with secure attachment and low avoidance style played freely and with a good, playful mood and were emotionally flexible and explorative. They used their body parts and personal space in a rich and relaxed way and openly displayed affects. In contrast, individuals who scored high on avoidance behavior scored low in both free and exploratory play.

11.1.2.4 Creative and Therapeutic Processes

Dance movement therapy appeals to the creative process as an integral part of its practice to facilitate self-awareness, change processes, and experience different ways of being in the world [12]. Even small changes in personal movement may offer the possibility of a new experiencing of oneself or another perspective on some worrying issue. That is, the individual may realize that there are other ways of being, of existing [10, 41].

The concept of procedural knowledge is key to understanding this idea. Dance movement therapy is interested in the meaning that comprises the experiences humans gather from early life through the ways they are cared for, physically held, and manipulated, as well as through the musicality of voices and sounds that surround them. This information shapes the experience of being with others and being oneself and is carried and kept into adult life. This is not conscious knowledge and it is different from the psychodynamic unconscious; however, it may be subject to psychodynamic issues, and this is what usually is met in the clinic. Rosenblatt [24] maintained that getting an insight is not enough: Besides restating interpretations, therapists need to think *with* the patient about creating ways to practice processes that affect the procedural structures. Due to its strong use of movement, dance, imagery, and metaphor and because it sometimes favors different states of consciousness, DMT touches the procedural memory/knowledge. This allows therapists not only to see its signs in the patients' movement and expressions, but also to open directions for change.

Further, movement for expression/dance are means for sublimation, manifestations of unspeakable contents (because of either repression or developmental or cognitive limitations). Movement/dance also may open the patient to identification, empathy, and experiencing body-movement mastery—aspects important for the relational sense of self in every client and certainly in psychiatric rehabilitation [10].

Carol Press [42] put forth an original and relevant approach to this issue. She integrated knowledge of dance, choreography, and psychoanalysis under a self-psychology perspective. Press mentioned that the close link between psychoanalysis and creative activity has been explored in the literature [42, 43] by comparing psychoanalysis with artistic work. In both, dreadful reminiscences, experiences, and imaginations are given form and meaning, and a deeper understanding of one's humanity is achieved. The restorative essence of creativity, therapy, and hope are linked closely to the concept of *trans-formation*, whose meaning in DMT is essentially twofold.

According to DMT's fundamental theoretical principle of embodiment, people are a felt and seen *form* who can *trans-form* themselves through movement and dance. Moreover, in the creative process, and especially in dance and other creative acts, the person engages in the aesthetic exploration of self-empathy and acceptance. Dance movement therapists hope that self-empathy and acceptance will grow in the patient; however, in many cases, the road to the patient experiencing such growth may be long. This model offers a specific perspective to the clinical phenomenon of "hiding the hope"—that is, hope's fragility, which can be perceived in some people. Press [44] maintained that healthy traits could be covered as a defense from feared attacks—a remnant from past disappointments—and thus weaken hope. According to Kohut [45], this is not a resistance but a self-preservation instinct. Creativity and psychotherapy allow for exploration and elaboration of *forward edge strivings*, giving *form to feelings and wishes* [44]. Although under-addressed, the idea of hope is cardinal for both mental health service users and professionals. Particularly for psychiatric rehabilitation, it is a fundamental principle of recovery.

Before presenting information about empirical research in psychiatric DMT, this section provides an interesting contribution of dance for health. Maraz et al. [46] inquired into the motivations of people who social dance for recreation and found three prevalent motives: mood enhancement, socializing, and escapism. *Mood enhancement* relates to the mood-improving and enlivening nature of dancing. *Socializing* connects to the experiences of being in good company and feeling affinity with the others. *Escapism* refers to the avoidance of emptiness, unpleasant mood, and average problems and is a motivation found also in persons with drug or alcohol addiction—thus, it can be supposed that dancing may be a healthy substitute. These three reasons for going dancing are reminiscent of DMT's proven main effects—anxiety and stress reduction.

11.2 Evidence on Dance Movement Therapy Interventions

Publications in peer-reviewed international journals about DMT in psychiatric rehabilitation are relatively scarce. One reason may be the lack of clarity concerning the practice of DMT in psychiatric settings (e.g., rehabilitation programs carried out in day care centers or in specific rehabilitation centers). In other areas of DMT research, scientific evidence has steadily grown over the last 50 years, gradually changing from qualitative reports towards empirical studies focused on outcomes of psychological health interventions. Koch et al. [47] identified only 1.3 studies per year published between 1996 and 2012 but witnessed significant global growth (6.8 studies/year) from 2012 to 2018. In their meta-analysis, Koch et al. analyzed 21 controlled intervention studies in DMT and 20 from other dance approaches, totaling 2374 individuals participating in dance-related activities.

The main topic of Koch et al.'s [47] work was the effects on psychological health. They analyzed randomized controlled trials in areas such as depression, anxiety, schizophrenia, autism, elderly patients, oncology, neurology, chronic heart failure, and cardiovascular disease, with special attention to the follow-up data available for eight studies. Overall, the available evidence on DMT outcomes regarded quality of life, clinical scorings (with specific subanalyses of depression and anxiety), interpersonal skills (the research area with the strongest positive evidence), and cognitive and psychomotor skills. Most of the DMT studies were conducted in settings oriented to preventing mental illnesses or in healthcare organizations with severely impaired patients. Overall, reported effects of DMT programs were small but of high clinical significance. They contributed to a consistent picture of DMT as achieving decreased anxiety and depression and generally improving quality of life and personal and cognitive skills. Longitudinal DMT studies tended to demonstrate that the observed effects remained stable or even increased over time.

11.2.1 Dance Movement Therapy Groups for Schizophrenia

Dance movement therapy has been implemented since the 1950s with people suffering from severe mental illness (SMI). Given the relative impact of medication on schizophrenia's negative symptoms, research in this area has aimed to investigate the influence of DMT in a controlled fashion. Martin et al. [48] recently reported on 44 patients randomly allocated in groups receiving 20 sessions of either DMT treatment or body psychotherapy (BPT), and a control group of 24 patients who received treatment as usual (TAU). The results relative to the intervention groups disclosed highly meaningful effects of both DMT and BPT on the severity of participants' negative symptoms (mean reduction of 20.6% in these clinical scorings).

Lee et al. [49] conducted a randomized trial to study DMT's influence on psychotic symptoms and affect in patients with schizophrenia. The DMT group ($n = 18$) attended 12 1-hour weekly sessions in addition to their regular medical treatment; the control group ($n = 20$) received only standard treatment. The intervention group obtained significant symptom reduction when compared with the control group. Several other investigations [50–52] also proved the positive effects of DMT for decreasing stress, facilitating stress management, and improving perceptions of well-being, positive affects, and body image, especially for affective symptomatology within the context of mental illness. In general, these studies present a positive image of the impact of DMT for schizophrenic syndromes and support including this modality in the treatment of persons with schizophrenia. In a mixed methods research [53], compared the treatment effects of a ten weeks group treatment with DMT on negative symptoms and psychosocial behavior of persons diagnosed with schizophrenia and another group in TAU. The qualitative outcomes indicate that participants in the DMT group felt more integrated, emotionally supported, improved their relationships and managed better their symptoms.

11.2.2 Dance Movement Therapy Groups for Depression

Karkou et al. [54] recently reviewed 817 studies focusing on the treatment of depression and reported the results of eight studies that met stringent inclusion criteria. Those eight encompassed 192 persons who received DMT as well as TAU and 159 who received TAU only. Two studies concerned patients with severe depression at the baseline, five related to patients with moderate depression, and one with a mild level of illness with adolescent girls in a mainstream school. These studies showed that DMT was associated with a diminution in the depression level: The groups whose patients began with severe depression decreased to a moderate level; others showed attenuation from a moderate to a mild level. In some studies, the effect was proven 3 months after the end of the treatment. The best effects were found in patients who underwent DMT and TAU simultaneously.

Of special interest within this field of investigation is a Cochrane review that focused on the impact of physical movement on depression. Rimer et al. [55] examined 39 studies encompassing 2326 subjects and demonstrated that exercise was similarly effective as antidepressants or psychological therapies in decreasing the symptoms of depression.

A further valuable example of the add-on effect of group DMT for depression is represented in the study Pylvänäinen et al. [56] conducted in an outpatient setting in Finland. The Finnish colleagues asked whether a DMT group intervention added to TAU more effectively eases depression symptoms when compared to TAU alone. Participants were adults with severe to moderate recurrent/chronic type depression; 12 of them received only TAU, and another 21 continued their TAU and added a 12-week DMT treatment. The Chace approach [57] was implemented together with aspects of Authentic Movement, including every group member's empathetic witnessing of the movement of other groups members and encouraging body and movement awareness. Pylvänäinen et al.'s [56] results presented a minimal depression level at the end of the project, probably meaning a full recovery, and indicated that DMT enhanced the TAU influence, as measured immediately after treatment and in a three-month follow-up. In a subsequent publication, Pylvänäinen [58] noted that 3 years later, the participants had not returned to the clinic.

To summarize, DMT has steadily demonstrated good results in well-designed studies whose major limitation was a small sample compared with research in other fields such as medicine. However, there is more research including larger numbers of participants, Hyvönen et al. [59], Pylvänäinen et al. [60].

11.3 Recovery in Mental Health and Dance Movement Therapy

Since the 1960s, major changes in mental health perceptions, policies, approaches, and practices have occurred, particularly in Western countries. The clinical viewpoint concerning the treatment of people with SMI also shifted in mental health research and the language used in the field. Currently, the worldwide accepted and evidence-based approach to psychiatric rehabilitation is *recovery*. Recovery mainly focuses on the personal journey of people coping with SMI [61] and stems from the needs of mental health service consumers to lead autonomous and fulfilling lives as part of society [62]. Many definitions of recovery have been proposed over the past decades. William Anthony [63], a pioneer in the field, described recovery as a "deeply personal, unique process of changing one's attitudes, values, feelings, goals, skills, and/or roles. It is a way of living a satisfying, hopeful, and contributing life even with limitations caused by illness" (p. 527). Other authors conceptualized recovery as a model or approach, whereas still others referred to it as an outcome [64]. A general scientific consensus is that recovery should be represented as a multidimensional paradigm that involves consideration of many aspects of life, including clinical, psychological, social, self-care, occupational, and environmental/contextual recovery [65, 66]. Fundamental recovery principles include hope, empowerment, choice, individualization, self-direction, purpose and meaning, awareness, integration, psychological well-being, shared decision-making, and healing [63, 64].

Dance movement therapy seems to be in full congruence with the recovery approach because it has similar core values and aims. The contribution of DMT is in using embodied techniques to enhance participants' well-being, integration, awareness, and function in all areas of life, as well as equipping them with tangible and effective coping skills to manage stress, change, and adaptation [67, 68].

With the movement towards inclusion of people experiencing mental illness in the general community, the scope of services and treatment opportunities has widened, as has the range of people pursuing mental health support. Recovery-oriented programs provide services in the areas of occupation, residence, education, and social inclusion [69]. Additionally, the importance of sustaining emotional support and opportunities for personal growth are acknowledged, and therefore programs generally offer recovery-oriented evidence-based interventions for individuals and groups. Those interventions are predominantly psychoeducational, cognitive behavioral therapy, and cognitive remediation based [70]; they do not use embodied techniques or creative expression methods.

Moreover, recovery-oriented groups tend to be highly heterogeneous. They consist of people experiencing a variety of psychiatric symptoms, at different severity levels, and with a range of communication, cognitive, and function abilities. The mental health literature noted some challenges pertaining to group work. These include participants' low motivation and disengagement, scarce attendance, high dropout rates, and issues caused by groups heterogeneity. The challenges are attributed, at least partially, to different treatment delivery methods and difficulty establishing a trusting therapeutic alliance [71]. Group DMT is adaptable to participants of all ages and abilities and offers alternative ways of obtaining and processing knowledge. The DMT session generally incorporates play, imagery, movement to music, and other topic-related expressive activities. Hence, DMT is suggested as an appropriate intervention to enhance participants' recovery processes.

Previous DMT research on people experiencing SMI was found to be highly effective in ameliorating psychological outcomes and functioning [54, 56, 72–74]. However, little has been explored about DMT's specific adaptability to the wider population seeking mental health care in the community (i.e., people in recovery who live in and are provided with psychiatric rehabilitation services in the community). One of the few evidences within this area of knowledge is a DMT qualitative study [75] that reported on adults coping with a range of diagnoses in an outpatient rehabilitation center in the United States. Its main aim was to evaluate whether a DMT and yoga therapy program contributed to participants' interpersonal skills and stress-management abilities. The 20-week program focused on self-expression, awareness, coping skills, stress reduction, and pro-social behavior. These foci represented desired recovery outcomes, although no mention of the term "recovery" was explicitly made. The program entailed mostly structured-movement experiences led by a dance movement therapist; the main interventions were breathing techniques, seated yoga postures, mirroring exercises, and activities based on Laban's and Bartenieff's fundamental DMT works.

Results indicated that participants recognized improvements in their ability to relax, as well as to incorporate newly obtained de-stressing techniques into their lives. Another relevant theme that emerged from the study was a growing awareness of patients' feelings and thoughts, linked to improved interpersonal relationships. Furthermore, all involved subjects found the group enjoyable and successful due to the creative movement and experiential activities, which differed from other didactic groups they had attended at the rehabilitation center. Over the past decade, a number of studies examined the contributions of other creative arts therapies to the recovery process [76–80]. This research confirmed the efficacy of arts therapies in contributing to participants' self-expression, sense of self-efficacy, presence, motivation, coping abilities, hope, and social recovery.

Melsom and Comins [81] discussed how therapists can apply DMT within the recovery framework. The clinically based constructs of the DMT-recovery model are empathy and a therapeutic movement relationship achieved by the use of movement and creativity, which foster participants' engagement, change processes, resilience, and hope. In DMT, participants find an opportunity to explore and express their experiences in personal and meaningful ways. This expression is achieved through body action, kinesthetic empathy, empathic reflection, symbolic movement expression, and other Chacean principles [57]. The DMT recovery model also applies the *transtheoretical model and stages of change* [82], an evidence-based model practiced in recovery work that stresses the importance of community-based work and adheres to the recovery framework [81]. However, this DMT recovery model has not been studied empirically. In conclusion, the movement-based group program seems to benefit people experiencing SMI because it provides tools to improve participants' well-being and social functioning in an experiential, embodied way that differs from other psychosocial programs.

11.4 A Field Experience: Recovery-Oriented Dance Movement Therapy

A recent empirical study [83] reported on a DMT-recovery intervention, a novel approach to DMT that combined with recovery principles to address the challenges of personal recovery and group heterogeneity. The Recovery-Oriented Dance Movement Therapy (RODMT) model was developed based on 15 years experience providing long-term DMT groups in several community-based mental health rehabilitation services in Israel and the United States. It applies specific recovery topics (such as symptom management) to DMT with the aim to make them more accessible, engaging, and meaningful to participants. Leading assumptions were that engaging in body-action activities might foster participants' learning of group topics and processing of personal themes, as well as enhance resonance and integration and, thus, contribute to participants' well-being. Additionally, participation in an enjoyable group, where self-expression and creativity are encouraged, was presumed to increase motivation to attend, socialization (one of the greatest challenges for people experiencing SMI), empowerment, hope, and self-determination. The main novelty of this approach is that no other recovery intervention focuses on mind–body integration or incorporates creative and expressive techniques to foster the recovery process. Furthermore, the psychotherapeutic components and unique DMT perspectives differentiate RODMT from other psychosocial and psychoeducational recovery interventions (Box 11.3).

Box 11.3 RODMT Basic Principles

Recovery-oriented dance movement therapy basic principles

- RODMT combines recovery principles and topics with the DMT approach and techniques
- Topics and themes derive from evidence-based recovery knowledge (e.g., illness management, psychosocial skill development, self-advocacy, hope, and self-determination) and group dynamics
- Body and movement-based activities may provide participants with personal meaning and a platform for creative expression and foster understanding, resonance, and integration of recovery topics
- DMT methods can contribute to participants' social and coping skills, such as stress and symptom reduction
- RODMT may provide an alternative and adaptive opportunity to obtain recovery content for participants with varying abilities and skills
- Suggested group structure consists of a movement warm-up (focus on awareness of self and others, bodily sensations, and introduction to the session's topic), central section (focus on a recovery topic and group themes through action-based activities), and closure (focus on embodiment and gathering of participants' experiences)

The RODMT intervention consisted of 13 structured sessions aiming at three essential recovery topics: developing social support, developing personal goals, and coping with stress. The RODMT session content was based on Mueser et al.'s [84] Illness Management and Recovery (IMR) workbook, from which discussion topics and questions were translated into movement-based activities congruent with recovery goals and outcomes. The sessions' structure included a movement-to-music warm-up leading to experiential activities related to the session topic, verbal processing of the group's experiences, and a movement group closure.

In addition to ongoing therapeutic goals such as developing body awareness and encouraging self-expression, each RODMT session has its own goals, depending on the topic being processed. The activities were carefully chosen with a clinical purpose and sensitivity to group dynamics. Other structural considerations were smooth and natural transitions between activities to foster a sense of safety, flow, and rhythm within each session, as well as throughout the course of the intervention.

The choice of activities or movement structure to use in the session considers the group's characteristics (such as participants' ages, abilities, and group dynamics) and developmental stage (Have safety and trust among participants been established? Are participants emotionally and cognitively ready to address a certain theme?); the therapist's philosophical and professional approach; and therapeutic alliance (Do the participants and therapist speak the same language? Do participants trust the therapist enough to "take risks" and delve into the theme being explored?). Emphasis was on participants' initiation of spontaneous movement, awareness of self and others, relational interaction, movement reflection and mirroring, imagery/symbolization, and individualization within the group dynamics.

Box 11.4 details the structure of a typical RODMT session (a group session with focus on the recovery topic *developing social support*, with middle-aged participants who were coping with SMI). The four goals of this specific session were those Mueser et al. [84] described, including (a) practice making connections, (b) define supportive relationships, (c) recognize the importance of social support, and (d) identify ways to increase it.

Box 11.4 A Typical RODMT Session Structure: Developing Social Support

Warm-up	The therapist chooses structures and movement activities that entail particular core DMT principles aimed at eliciting therapeutic processes. Group DMT sessions begin in a circle with a movement-to-music warm-up. The warm-up consists of spontaneous movements led by the participants and reinforced by the therapist—such as stretching different body parts, breathing, and dancing—that adhere to the DMT principles of self-expression, group synchrony, cohesion, and symbolism. The aims of all DMT warm-ups are to set the group environment; check in with participants, helping them gain presence, awareness, and a sense of grounding (be in the "here and now," be aware of bodily sensations, and focus); make connections among group members; support a sense of belonging; and bring the group to a cohesiveness that would allow for the theme exploration The emphasis in this example warm-up is ensuring eye contact is made among all participants and that everyone is acknowledged in some way. Participants are requested to present themselves through a movement that would illustrate something they would like to share about themselves (How you are feeling today? Show something you enjoy doing). The rest of the group witnesses (acknowledges) each member's gesture and responds to him or her by repeating their name and movement. This experiential activity encourages, among other things, communication, listening skills, ability to see the other, feeling seen and recognized, empathy, practice making eye contact, and observation, which are essential for building healthy relationships. In the context of the session's topic, this activity challenges participants' decisions on how they would choose to present themselves and which parts of themselves they would expose or share
Core	According to Schmais [85], each specific DMT group therapeutic factor (i.e., expression, synchrony/cohesion, vitalization, education, integration, and symbolism) are addressed within the sessions. Use of symbolic movement expression (e.g., embodying a feeling instead of just saying it) is believed to bridge the participant's inner and outer worlds. Additionally, the use of symbolism and images fosters creativity To foster social support, the therapist uses a prop made of long, colorful fabric strips tied to a ring shaped like a sun. in turn, each participant takes a strip and says what social support means to him or her. At the end of the round, the "sun of social support" is held by all participants, and the therapist summarizes the qualities of a supportive relationship: respectful, reciprocal, accepting, fun, helpful, and so forth. 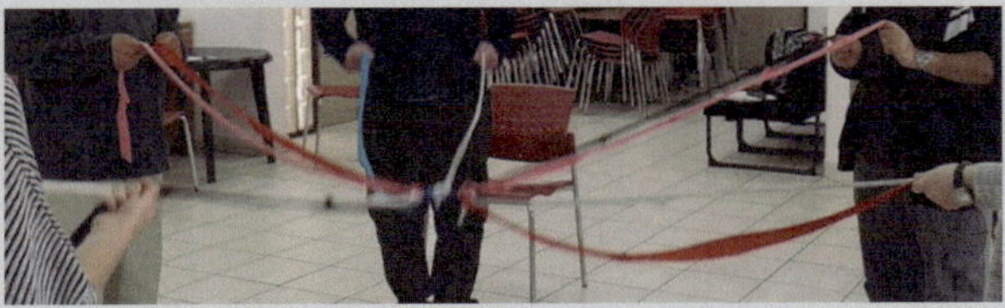

	The next nonverbal activity is meant to explore different types of relationships and increase awareness of the experience of being in them. The instruction is for two participants at a time to meet in the center of the circle and respond or react without words to a sentence the facilitator offers. Examples include meeting a close friend who you have not seen for a long time, meeting a stranger, meeting someone who gets down on you all the time, or meeting someone with whom who you feel comfortable, accepted, and equal in the relationship The therapist looks for and encourages exaggerated movement expression that would bring forth feelings such as shyness, embarrassment, hesitance, excitement, rejection, passion, or warmness. The associations among feelings, personal experience, and life situations are continuously reflected back to participants to foster mind–body connection, integration, and resonance (personal meaning and embodiment) The group then verbally processes the experiences from the activity. Participants could share and reflect on relationships they had in their own lives, relate to whether they were supportive or whether they wanted to examine them further and possibly change something, and discuss the value of maintaining supportive relationships Once the importance of having a supportive relationship is established, the practical questions come—How to increase social support? How to make connections? The facilitator passes a ball in the group. Each participant holds the ball and offers solutions, such as meeting and talking to new people or strengthening existing relationships, and ideas on how to initiate conversations (e.g., creating eye contact, smiling, "opening lines" and "icebreakers," and conversation topics). Then, that participant tosses the ball to the next participant
	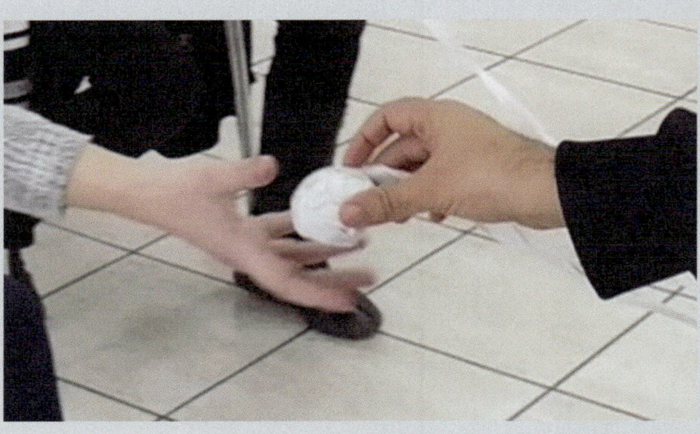
	The ball toss is active (engagement); it involves the use of strength (vitality) and directiveness (clear focus and intention). This activity may lead to a deeper movement and verbal exploration of important themes such as boundaries, exposure, intimacy, and personal barriers to relationships This session focuses on *evaluating* relationships. The following sessions provide opportunities to *practice* social skills using movement activities such as mirroring to increase empathy and awareness of others (as discussed earlier in this chapter), spontaneous movement initiation games to encourage spontaneity—a necessary skill for having a conversation, and bodily enactment of personal traits that participants would like to bring forth in their relationships

Closing	The central part of the sessions often raises emotions, questions, and uncertainties. For this reason, it is especially important to end the group with a settling experience. An example closure activity could be passing an imaginary object around the circle through movement. For example, pass an imaginary energy ball into which each participant injects a quality, feeling, image, or learning they took from the session and want to pass to the rest of the group. In the closure, the therapist reflects back to the group any observations and collective insights from the session and communicates main points of the topic discussed 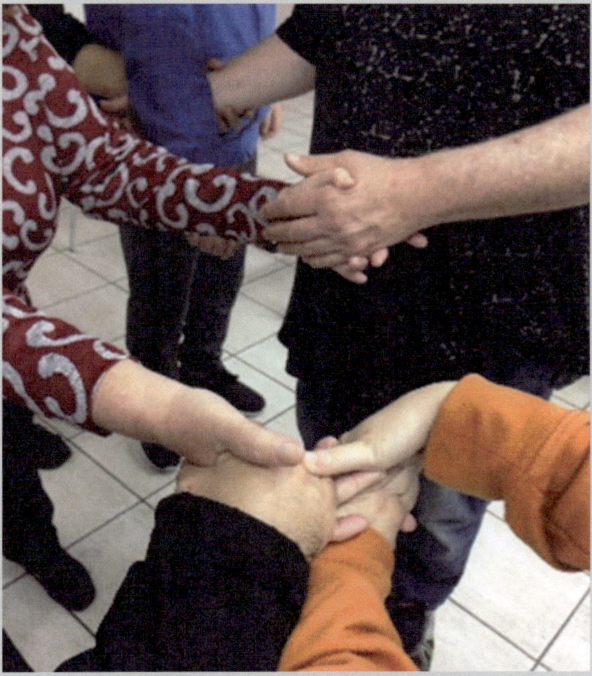
Roles	• The RODMT facilitator's role is to help participants process the knowledge they acquire from the movement experience and tie it to daily life experiences. In addition, the facilitator reflects back to the group (using verbal and nonverbal techniques) any observed connections between participants' experiences, which enhances a sense of belonging and self-worth • The role of the group participants is to support, witness, reflect, and empower one another to express and share their experiences

The RODMT intervention took place in nine recovery-oriented community-based services in Israel over 6 months (from September 2018 to February 2019). It involved 98 participants assigned to either a 13-week RODMT group or an active control group that received the equivalent topics using the IMR workbook. Groups were led by qualified DMT or IMR facilitators (not the researcher). Standardized surveys, the Illness Management and Recovery Scale (IMRS), and the Patient Activation Measure (PAM) were administered before and after the intervention to assess participants' engagement and recovery. Knowledge questionnaires about coping with stress and developing social support were administered before and after their respective topic sessions to compare knowledge gain between groups. Additionally, the researcher interviewed five RODMT participants regarding their overall experiences from the group [83].

Data analyses indicated no significant differences between groups in the parameters checked (participants of RODMT and IMR groups had similar dropout rates and results in recovery measures, personal-activation level, and knowledge obtained in the groups). A thematic analysis of the interviews revealed that participants' experiences of the RODMT were positive. They described the group as "enjoyable," "nice," "interesting," and "pleasant" and said they felt supported in the group. Participants especially talked about enjoying the experiential activities and gave examples of mind–body connections they made, relating a specific movement experience to a feeling or insight. Three participants said they gained awareness from the group and gave examples of applying stress reduction strategies they learned in the group to their daily lives. Because both RODMT and the established recovery intervention IMR had similar impact on participants' recovery, the researcher suggests that RODMT can serve as an appropriate intervention in the recovery framework for people coping with SMI [83]. Further research is still needed to establish the efficacy of RODMT, also in different settings and in larger patient samples.

11.5 Future Directions

Dance movement therapy derives from a wide range of psychological and philosophical paradigms. Each dance movement therapist brings unique perspectives into their work. Some draw more heavily on psychological roots, some come with a dance-based orientation, and others incorporate neuroscientific understandings. However, all share and practice the fundamental principles of DMT as described in this chapter. Verbal or written descriptions and explanations cannot provide a full picture of what happens in a DMT session. The kinesthetic and other sensorial and emotional experiences that occur cannot be conveyed through words. Further, the sessions differ from one population to another (e.g., a session with children on the autism spectrum will not look like a session for adults with SMI) and between individual and group work.

As previously discussed, research in DMT is gradually accumulating and its applications in various mental health subfields are growing as well. Evidence has been demonstrated for the effectiveness of DMT with people experiencing SMI but is still lacking on DMT in mental health rehabilitation and recovery. Different definitions of mental health services and settings around the world make it difficult to assess how widespread DMT is in mental health rehabilitation or what therapists emphasize in their work with people coping with SMI.

The authors of this chapter feel that it is important for dance movement therapists to learn the "recovery language" and stay updated on current mental health approaches so they can convey DMT's advantages in enhancing the integration of core recovery topics. Because mental health rehabilitation practices are evidence-based, it is necessary to demonstrate the applicability of DMT to the recovery processes through more research. The RODMT study [83] highlighted in this chapter addressed the gap between DMT practice and mental health rehabilitation research and offered a novel perspective to practicing dance movement therapists.

This chapter introduced DMT in psychiatry and clarified some DMT core principles and benefits of practicing it in psychiatric rehabilitation. The authors intended to emphasize the adaptability of DMT to diverse groups of people in need of mental health services; the opportunity it provides participants to express themselves through creative means, gain knowledge, and process information through body action; and to stress the correspondence between DMT and recovery paradigms.

References

1. American Dance Therapy Association. What is dance/movement therapy? 2019. https://adta.org/clinical-info-sheets/. Accessed 15 Oct 2019.
2. Wosien MG. Sacred dance: encounter with the gods. New York: Thames and Hudson; 1974.
3. Chaiklin S. We dance from the moment our feet touch the earth. In: Chaiklin S, Wengrower H, editors. The art and science of dance movement therapy: life is dance. New York: Routledge; 2016. p. 3–11.
4. Bynum B. Tarantism. Lancet. 2001;358:1736. https://doi.org/10.1016/S0140-6736(01)06731-9.
5. Hobbs K, compiler. Isadora Duncan dance video [video file]. 2013 Jun 13. https://www.youtube.com/watch?v=rkr_h0jlo7A. Accessed 8 Nov 2019.
6. Mooiman M, compiler. The witch [video file]. 2014 Jun 23. https://wwwyoutubecom/watch?v=AtLSSuFlJ5c. 20 Sept 2018.
7. Miranda R. Introduction. In: Fernandes C, editor. O corpo en movimiento. Sao Paulo: Annablume; 2000. p. 17–21.
8. Laban R, Ullman L, editors. The mastery of movement. Boston: Plays; 1971.
9. Ullman L, editor. Rudolf Laban speaks about movement and dance: lectures and articles. Addlestone: Laban Art of Movement Centre; 1971.
10. Wengrower H. The creative–artistic process in dance movement therapy. In: Chaiklin S, Wengrower H, editors. The art and science of dance movement therapy: life is dance. New York: Routledge; 2016. p. 13–32.
11. Darwin C. The expression of emotion in man and animals. New York: D. Appleton; 1872–1899. http://www.gutenberg.org/files/1227/1227-h/1227-h.htm. Accessed 20 Dec 2019.
12. Stanton Jones K. Dance movement therapy in psychiatry. London: Routledge; 1992.
13. Levy F. Dance/movement therapy: a healing art. Rev. ed. Reston: American Alliance for Health, Physical Education, Recreation and Dance; 1992.
14. Chaiklin S. Marian Chace: dancer & pioneer dance therapist. In Marian Chace biography. American Dance Therapy Association. 2019. https://adta.org/marian-chace-biography/. Accessed 8 Nov 2019.

15. Sandel S. The process of empathic reflection in dance therapy. In: Sandel S, Chaiklin S, Lohn A, editors. Foundations of dance movement therapy: the life and work of Marian Chace. Columbia: Marian Chace Memorial Fund of the American Dance Therapy Association; 1993. p. 98–111.
16. Wengrower H. I am here to move and dance with you: dance movement therapy with autism syndrome disorder. In: Karkou V, editor. Arts therapies in schools: research and practice. London: Jessica Kingsley; 2010. p. 179–97.
17. Iacoboni M. Imitation, empathy, and mirror neurons. Annu Rev Psychol. 2009;60:653–70. https://doi.org/10.1146/annurev.psych.60.110707.163604.
18. Anzieu D. El Yo-Piel [The skin ego]. Vidarrazaga Zimmermann S, translator. Madrid: Biblioteca Nueva; 1989/1998.
19. Caldwell C. Bodyfulness. Boulder: Shambala; 2018.
20. Winnicott DW. Psycho-somatic illness in its positive and negative aspects. Int J Psychoanal. 1966;47:510–6.
21. Chaiklin S, Wengrower H. Introduction. In: Chaiklin S, Wengrower H, editors. The art and science of dance movement therapy: life is dance. New York: Routledge; 2016. p. xxix–xxxii.
22. Tortora S. Dance/movement psychotherapy in early childhood treatment and in pediatric oncology. In: Chaiklin S, Wengrower H, editors. The art and science of dance movement therapy: life is dance. New York: Routledge; 2016. p. 159–81.
23. Damasio A. The feeling of what happens: body and emotion in the making of consciousness. New York: Harcourt Brace; 1999.
24. Rosenblatt A. Insight, working through, and practice: the role of procedural knowledge. J Am Psychoanal Assoc. 2004;52:189–207. https://doi.org/10.1177/00030651040520011901.
25. Fuchs T, Koch SC. Embodied affectivity: on moving and being moved. Front Psychol. 2014;5:508. https://doi.org/10.3389/fpsyg.2014.00508.
26. Gallagher S. How the body shapes the mind. Oxford: Oxford University Press; 2005.
27. Thompson E. Empathy and consciousness. J Conscious Stud. 2001;8:1–32.
28. Fischman D. Therapeutic relationships and kinesthetic empathy. In: Chaiklin S, Wengrower H, editors. The art and science of dance movement therapy: life is dance. New York: Routledge; 2016. p. 33–52.
29. Mehling WE, Wrubel J, Daubenmier JJ, Price CJ, Kerr CE. Body awareness: a phenomenological inquiry into the common ground of mindbody therapies. Philos Ethics Humanit Med. 2011;6:6. https://doi.org/10.1186/1747-5341-6-6.
30. Shafir T. Using movement to regulate emotion: neurophysiological findings and their application in psychotherapy. Front Psychol. 2016;7:1451. https://doi.org/10.3389/fpsyg.2016.01451.
31. Damasio A. Mental self: the person within. Nature. 2003;423:227. https://doi.org/10.1038/423227a.
32. Pollatos O, Gramann K, Schandry R. Neural systems connecting interoceptive awareness and feelings. Hum Brain Mapp. 2007;28:9–18. https://doi.org/10.1002/hbm.20258.
33. Critchley HD, Wiens S, Rotshtein P, Öhman A, Dolan RJ. Neural systems supporting interoceptive awareness. Nat Neurosci. 2004;7:189–95.
34. Fujino H. Body awareness and mental health: a body psychotherapy case study. Body Mov Dance Psychother. 2016;11:249–62. https://doi.org/10.1080/17432979.2016.1150882.
35. Hindi FS. How attention to interoception can inform dance/movement therapy. Am J Dance Ther. 2012;34:129–40.
36. Ardizzi M, Ambrosecchia M, Buratta L, Ferri F, Peciccia M, Donnari S, et al. Interoception and positive symptoms in schizophrenia. Front Hum Neurosci. 2016;10:379. https://doi.org/10.3389/fnhum.2016.00379.
37. White QE. Laban's movement theories: a dance/movement therapist's perspective. In: Chaiklin S, Wengrower H, editors. The art and science of dance movement therapy: life is dance. New York: Routledge; 2016. p. 235–54.
38. Loman S, Sossin M. Kestenberg movement profile in dance/movement therapy: an introduction. In: Chaiklin S, Wengrower H, editors. The art and science of dance movement therapy: life is dance. New York: Routledge; 2016. p. 255–84.

39. Sossin KM. Musings on theoretical and research contributions of the KMP within the context of nonverbal studies. In: Kestenberg Amighi J, Loman S, Sossin KM, editors. The meaning of movement: embodied developmental, clinical, and cultural perspectives of the Kestenberg movement profile. New York: Routledge; 2018. p. 237–317.
40. Feniger-Schaal R, Hart Y, Lotan N, Koren-Karie N, Noy L. The body speaks: using the mirror game to link attachment and non-verbal behavior. Front Psychol. 2018;9:1560. https://doi.org/10.3389/fpsyg.2018.01560.
41. Wengrower, H. Dance comes to the front stage in dance movement therapy. In Wengrower, H. Chaiklin, S., editors. Dance and creativity within dance movement therapy. International perspectives. New York: Routledge; 2021. pp. 9–24.
42. Press CM. Restoration of hope: the creation of a dance. Psychoanal Inq. 2006;26:407–21. https://doi.org/10.2513/s07351690pi2603_8.
43. Hagman G. Aesthetic experience: beauty, creativity, and the search for the ideal. New York: Rodopi; 2005. p. 122.
44. Press CM. Psychoanalysis, creativity, and hope: forward edge strivings in the life and work of choreographer Paul Taylor. J Am Acad Psychoanal Dyn Psychiatry. 2005;33:119–36. https://doi.org/10.1521/jaap.33.1.119.65884.
45. Kohut H. How does analysis cure? Chicago: University of Chicago Press; 1984.
46. Maraz A, Király O, Urbán R, Griffiths MD, Demetrovics Z. Why do you dance? Development of the dance motivation inventory (DMI). PLoS One. 2015;10:e0122866. https://doi.org/10.1371/journal.pone.0122866.
47. Koch SC, Riege RFF, Tisborn K, Biondo J, Martin L, Beelmann A. Effects of dance movement therapy and dance on health-related psychological outcomes: a meta-analysis update. Front Psychol. 2019;10:1806. https://doi.org/10.3389/fpsyg.2019.01806.
48. Martin L, Koch S, Hirjak D, Fuchs T. Overcoming disembodiment: the effect of movement therapy on negative symptoms in schizophrenia; a multicenter randomized controlled trial. Front Psychol. 2016a;7:483. https://doi.org/10.3389/fpsyg.2016.00483.
49. Lee HJ, Jang SH, Lee SY, Hwang KS. Effectiveness of dance/movement therapy on affect and psychotic symptoms in patients with schizophrenia. Arts Psychother. 2015;45:64–8. https://doi.org/10.1016/j.aip.2015.07.003.
50. Bräuninger I. Specific dance movement therapy interventions–which are successful? An intervention and correlation study. Arts Psychother. 2014;41:445–57. https://doi.org/10.1016/j.aip.2014.08.002.
51. Jeong YJ, Hong SC, Lee MS, Park MC, Kim YK, Suh CM. Dance movement therapy improves emotional responses and modulates neurohormones in adolescents with mild depression. Int J Neurosci. 2005;115:1711–20.
52. Koch S, Kunz T, Lykou S, Cruz R. Effects of dance movement therapy and dance on health-related psychological outcomes: a meta-analysis. Arts Psychother. 2014;41:46–64. https://doi.org/10.1016/j.aip.2013.10.004.
53. Bryl K, Bradt J, Cechnicki A, Fisher K, Sossin KM, Goodill S. The role of dance/movement therapy in the treatment of negative symptoms in schizophrenia: a mixed methods pilot study. J Ment Health. 2020. https://doi.org/10.1080/09638237.2020.1757051.
54. Karkou V, Aithal S, Zubala A, Meekums B. Effectiveness of dance movement therapy in the treatment of adults with depression: a systematic review with meta-analyses. Front Psychol. 2019;10:936. https://doi.org/10.3389/fpsyg.2019.00936.
55. Rimer J, Dwan K, Lawlor DA, Greig CA, McMurdo M, Morley W, et al. Exercise for depression. Cochrane Database Syst Rev. 2012;7:CD004366. https://doi.org/10.1002/14651858.CD004366.pub5.
56. Pylvänäinen PM, Muotka JS, Lappalainen R. A dance movement therapy group for depressed adult patients in a psychiatric outpatient clinic: effects of the treatment. Front Psychol. 2015;6:980. https://doi.org/10.3389/fpsyg.2015.00980.
57. Chaiklin S, Schmais C. The Chace approach to dance therapy. In: Sandel S, Chaiklin S, Lohn A, editors. Foundations of dance/movement therapy: the life and work of Marian Chace. Columbia, MD: Marian Chace Memorial Fund; 1993. p. 75–97.

58. Pylvänäinen PM. Embodied treatment of depression: the development of a dance movement therapy model. In: Zubala A, Karkou V, editors. Arts therapies in the treatment of depression. New York: Routledge; 2018. p. 120–36.
59. Hyvönen K, Pylvänäinen PM, Muotka J and Lappalainen R. The effects of dance movement therapy in the treatment of depression: A multicenter, randomized control trial in Finland. Front Psychol. 2020;11:1687. https://doi.org/10.3389/fpsyg.2020.01687.
60. Pylvänäinen P, Hyvönen K and Muotka J. The profiles of body image associate with changes in depression among participants in dance movement therapy group. Front Psychol. 2020;11:564788. https://doi.org/10.3389/fpsyg.2020.564788.
61. Deegan PE. Recovery: the lived experience of rehabilitation. Psychosoc Rehabil J. 1988;11: 11–9. https://doi.org/10.1037/h0099565.
62. Onken SJ, Craig CM, Ridgway P, Ralph RO, Cook JA. An analysis of the definitions and elements of recovery: a review of the literature. Psychiatr Rehabil J. 2007;31:9–22. https://doi.org/10.2975/31.1.2007.9.22.
63. Anthony WA. Recovery from mental illness: the guiding vision of the mental health service system in the 1990s. Psychol Rehabil J. 1993;16:11–23. https://doi.org/10.1037/h0095655.
64. Corrigan PW, Ralph RO. Introduction: recovery as consumer vision and research paradigm. In: Ralph RO, Corrigan PW, editors. Recovery in mental illness: broadening our understanding of wellness. Washington, DC: American Psychological Association; 2005. p. 3–17.
65. Lal S. Prescribing recovery as the new mantra for mental health: does one prescription serve all? Can J Occup Ther. 2010;77:82–9. https://doi.org/10.2182/cjot.2010.77.2.4.
66. Ramon S. The place of social recovery in mental health and related services. Int J Environ Res Public Health. 2018;15:1052. https://doi.org/10.3390/ijerph15061052.
67. Bräuninger I. The efficacy of dance movement therapy group on improvement of quality of life: a randomized controlled trial. Arts Psychother. 2012;39:296–303. https://doi.org/10.1016/j.aip.2012.03.008.
68. Cruz RF. Dance/movement therapy and developments in empirical research: the first 50 years. Am J Dance Ther. 2016;38:297–302. https://doi.org/10.1007/s10465-016-9224-2.
69. Slade M, Amering M, Farkas M, Hamilton B, O'Hagan M, Panther G, et al. Uses and abuses of recovery: implementing recovery-oriented practices in mental health systems. World Psychiatry. 2014;13:12–20. https://doi.org/10.1002/wps.20084.
70. Morin L, Franck N. Rehabilitation interventions to promote recovery from schizophrenia: a systematic review. Front Psych. 2017;128:100. https://doi.org/10.3389/fpsyt.2017.00100.
71. Fernandez E, Salem D, Swift JK, Ramtahal N. Meta-analysis of dropout from cognitive behavioral therapy: magnitude, timing, and moderators. J Consult Clin Psychol. 2015;83:1108–22. https://doi.org/10.1037/ccp0000044.
72. Martin L, Pohlmann V, Koch S, Fuchs T. Back into life: effects of embodied therapies on patients with schizophrenia. Eur Psychother. 2016b;13:179–94.
73. Priebe S, Savill M, Wykes T, Bentall RP, Reininghaus U, Lauber C, et al. Effectiveness of group body psychotherapy for negative symptoms of schizophrenia: multicentre randomised controlled trial. Br J Psychiatry. 2016;209:54–61. https://doi.org/10.1192/bjp.bp.115.171397.
74. Punkanen M, Saarikallio S, Luck G. Emotions in motion: short-term group form dance/movement therapy in the treatment of depression; a pilot study. Arts Psychother. 2014;41:493–7. https://doi.org/10.1016/j.aip.2014.07.001.
75. Barton EJ. Movement and mindfulness: a formative evaluation of a dance/movement and yoga therapy program with participants experiencing severe mental illness. Am J Dance Ther. 2011;33:157–81. https://doi.org/10.1007/s10465-011-9121-7.
76. Allan J, Barford H, Horwood F, Stevens J, Tanti G. ATIC: developing a recovery-based art therapy practice. Int J Art Ther. 2015;20:1427. https://doi.org/10.1080/17454832.2014.968597.
77. McCaffrey T, Edwards J, Fannon D. Is there a role for music therapy in the recovery approach in mental health? Arts Psychother. 2011;38:185–9. https://doi.org/10.1016/j.aip.2011.04.006.
78. Papagiannaki A, Shinebourne P. The contribution of creative art therapies to promoting mental health: using interpretative phenomenological analysis to study therapists' understandings of working with self-stigmatisation. Arts Psychother. 2016;50:66–74. https://doi.org/10.1016/j.aip.2016.06.007.

79. Spandler H, Secker J, Kent L, Hacking S, Shenton J. Catching life: the contribution of arts initiatives to recovery approaches in mental health. J Psychiatr Ment Health Nurs. 2007;14:791–9. https://doi.org/10.1111/j.1365-2850.2007.01174.x.
80. Van Lith T. Art making as a mental health recovery tool for change and coping. Art Ther. 2015;32:5–12. https://doi.org/10.1080/07421656.2015.992826.
81. Melsom AM, Comins J. A dance/movement therapy recovery model. In: Neilsen F, King R, Baker F, editors. Creative arts in counseling and mental health. London: Sage; 2016. p. 122–33.
82. Prochaska J, DiClemente C. Stages and processes of self-change of smoking: toward an integrative model of change. Consult Clin Psychol. 1983;51:390–5. https://doi.org/10.1037//0022-006X.51.3.390.
83. Bendel-Rozow T. Recovery-oriented dance movement therapy: a controlled trial in mental health rehabilitation (Order No. 27833628). Available from Dissertations & Theses @ Lesley university; ProQuest Dissertations & Theses Global. (2395299920). 2020. Retrieved from https://digitalcommons.lesley.edu/expressive_dissertations/98/.
84. Mueser KT, Corrigan PW, Hilton DW, Tanzman B, Schaub A, Gingerich S, et al. Illness management and recovery: a review of the research. Psychiatr Serv. 2002;53:1272–84. https://doi.org/10.1176/appi.ps.53.10.1272.
85. Schmais C. Healing processes in group dance therapy. Am J Dance Ther. 1985;8:17. https://doi.org/10.1007/BF02251439.

Training Standard of Dance Movement Therapy in E.U. and Italian Contribution to Research on Recovery

12

Sara Diamare

Wengrower and Bendel-Rozow start from a strong theoretical construct in support of the use of DMT in mental health.

They propose a very interesting model for implementing research in the field of psychiatric rehabilitation with a view to recovery. In addition, they provide a meta-analysis of mental health research with DMT, in particular in the USA and Israel.

In many EU countries, DMT is unfortunately not legally recognized. In psychiatric rehabilitation settings [1], the dance therapist, if not already specialized in psychotherapy, can act only as part of a team with a healthcare figure. DMT is also integrated as a therapeutic strategy in a psychotherapy setting if performed by a psychotherapist doctor/psychologist.

The Italian Professional Dance Movement Therapy Association DMT-APID® (www.apid.it), established [2] on the 27th October 1997 in order to promote, support and protect the professional, ethical and scientific level of Dance Movement Therapy's quality and to create a community of DMT professionals, is one of the founding member (2007), together with Germany, Greece, Hungary, Latvia, The Netherlands, Poland, Russia, Spain and UK, of the European Association Dance Movement Therapy. The EADMT (www.eadmt.com), represents national professional DMT associations in Europe (including Israel), is working actively to promote the development of professional practice and the legal recognition of the profession.

Being the DMT's method still not legally recognized so as not widespread in E.U, it is often confused with playful animation activities, that is why it is appropriate to clarify the dividing line between the use of dance as exercise and the use of DMT as recovery or as psychotherapy. In Italy, there are also experiments being carried out on the use of recreational dance performed in pairs or in groups for their socializing dimension [3].

S. Diamare (✉)
Local Health Unit, Naples 1 Centre, DMT—A.P.I.D.®, Naples, Italy

U. Volpe (ed.), *Arts Therapies in Psychiatric Rehabilitation*,
https://doi.org/10.1007/978-3-030-76208-7_12

But the way in which DMT helps a psychotic patient explore the healthy parts of their inner life shows that it has a specifically defined role to play in the psychiatric rehabilitation setting—and consequently so does the professional figure who provides the service.

Any psychotherapeutic process may lead to the re-emergence of a patient's inner ghosts. Consequently, it is clear that DMT must entail specific training so that the uncontrolled emergence of drives can be avoided.

The reflection that follows is that dance, as a structured motor activity, offers a playful dimension to treatment with effects on mood and socialization. DMT then emerges as rehabilitation, as psychotherapy or as a transformative formula proposed to the psychiatric team by personnel who are adequately trained in DMT.

The discovery of mirror neurons [4] has made it possible to understand the neurofunctional mechanisms underlying the imitation of human behaviour and learning by gestural codes.

As proposed by H. Wengrower and T. Bendel-Rozow, the mirroring that is often used in DMT to promote empathy can become a central experience for psychodynamic and relational research. The imitation and learning of new gestural and behavioural codes allows a person to expand their palette of emotional expressiveness and to explore the moods related to those codes. From this perspective, DMT offers an appropriate ground for psychiatric rehabilitation.

In Italy, and precisely by Local Health Unit Naples 1 Centre, C.O.U. Quality & Humanization, we are also conducting a pilot study with the "mirror game" to see the extent to which it can activate a path of psycho-corporative empowerment. In particular, we started an analysis on 120 subjects belonging to homogeneous groups [5] in training contexts.

A self-assessment form [6, 7] in simple and shareable language was used in order to demonstrate an internal construct validity [8]. The adoption of this form is also being studied in psychiatric settings both for the assessment of movement and to support empowerment processes, which are considered vital for patients, operators and caregivers.

In this case, the aim of DMT contributes towards not only the rehabilitation of the psychiatric patient but also the improvement of the treatment setting and its systems of interaction with the patient.

Wengrower and Bendel-Rozow argue that in psychiatric rehabilitation the hope of "healing" can be weak in the experience of the operator and the patient, so it becomes problematic to set up a shared project. In our opinion, the DMT model, implying the integration of the 'different' into the group/community through the adoption of gestural codes and common rhythms, can lead to transformation [8, 9] in an inclusive environment. At the base of this assumption is the scientific trans-theoretical construct of Prochaska and DiClemente which, as highlighted by Wengrower and Bendel-Rozow, introduces the concept of the stages of change in community-based work that adheres to the recovery framework [10].

Relational maternage models [11] of the patient's team and community, based on creative and motor exchange, can become part of the operator's ongoing training and the setting's cross-discipline training (dance therapy/art therapy). Such training allows the exploration of new relational codes to the family (family dance therapy) and within it to the patient himself or herself.

The process of transformation allows us to understand that change is always possible through interaction and reciprocity. This is also described in action-research modules on formulas for the reception of migrants, who in many parts of Italy have become experimental prototypes of local management of social policies [12, 13].

An environment of inclusion, where professionally updated training modules in DMT for psychiatric operators directly intersect with DMT courses for psychiatric patients and caregivers—thereby allowing for the sharing of ideas—can transform the community into one where hope is placed not exclusively in the resolution of the individual, but in the interaction of the group.

In conclusion, Wengrower and Bendel-Rozow skilfully and methodically open the way to scientific discussion and stimulate questions on how to collect data in the psychiatric field. The impulse intended to be given to research in this area is supported by the validity of the illustrated theoretical construct. Scientific research can also support the institutional and formal recognition processes of the DMT figure in all EU countries.

References

1. Volpe U, Facchini D, Magnotti R, Diamare S, Denti E, Viganò CA. Le arti-terapie nel contesto della riabilitazione psicosociale in Italia: una rassegna critica. Psichiatria e Psicoterapia. 2016;35(4):154–80. https://www.fioritieditore.com/wp-content/uploads/2017/04/03Volpeeta l.2016_04PP.pdf.
2. APID Consiglio Direttivo (cur) "Vent'anni di APID". In: ilmiolibro self publishing collana La community; 2018. ISBN Libro: 9788892341593.
3. Tavormina R, Tavormina MGM, Nemoianni E. Dance and go on: a project of psychosocial rehabilitation on the road. Psychiatria Danubina. 2015;27(Suppl. 1):143–7.
4. Gallese V. Embodied simulation: from neurons to phenomenal experience. Phenomenol Cogn Sci. 2005;4:23–48.
5. Diamare S, et al. Un metodo di Embodied Education in Riabilitazione: approcci di valutazione partecipata e di empowerment psicocorporeo. J Adv Health Care. 2019; https://doi.org/10.36017/jahc1909-002.
6. D'Ambrosio M, Diamare S, Furia R, Nappi B, Ruocco C, Salerno M. La Metodologia Embodied per le disabilità sensoriali. Res Trends Humanit Educ Philos. 2019. http://www.rth.unina.it/index.php/rth/issue/view/453.
7. Diamare S. Per la valutazione del percorso di tras-formazione nell'ottica salutogenica. In: Teatro come metodologia trasformativa, La scena educativa fatta ad arte. Tra ricerca e formazione, a cura di D'Ambrosio M., Cartografie pedagogiche, Ed. Liguori; 2016.
8. Diamare S, Ferrara A, Ricciardi O, Verniti S. Direzionalità e condensazione del movimento corporeo attraverso uno strumento di autovalutazione. Phenomena J. 2020; https://doi.org/10.32069/pj.2020.1.64.
9. Tavormina R, Diamare S, D'Alterio V, Nappi B, Ruocco C, Guida E. Development of the life skills for promotion of health with art-therapy. Int Psychiatria Danubina. 2014;26(Suppl. 1):167–72.
10. Margrethe MA, Jill C. Chapter 11: A dance/movement therapy recovery model engagement in stages of change. In: Creative arts in counseling and mental health. London: Sage. 2016; https://doi.org/10.4135/9781506306049.

11. Ferenczi S. Le tappe evolutive del senso di realtà. In: Fondamenti di Psicoanalisi, Guaraldi; 1972.
12. Mignosi E. Dance movement therapy in educational training for intercultural experiences. In: Hougham R, Pitruzzella S, Scoble S, editors. Cultural landscapes in the arts therapies. Plymouth: University of Plymouth Press; 2017. p. 187–205. ISBN 978-1-84102-424-0.
13. Mignosi E. Bridges between people: nonverbal mediation in an intercultural perspective and training proposals. Studi sulla Formazione. 2019;21:259–75. https://doi.org/10.13128/Studi_Formaz-25569. ISSN 2036-6981.

Dance Movement Therapy as an Alternative for Rehabilitating People with Mental Disorders

13

Juanjuan Ren, Chenyu Ye, and Chen Zhang

In this chapter, the authors thoroughly reviewed the development history of dance movement therapy (DMT), the procedure of clinical application, the effect of different population, and the outlook for the future in a concise language.

DMT can be viewed as a form of psychotherapy that uses movement and dance to further people's emotional, cognitive, physical, and social integration [1]. It is an interdisciplinary product combining medicine, psychology, and art. In the treatment process, DMT emphasizes the spontaneity of movement and focuses on self-expression. People communicate conscious and unconscious feelings through physical development and creative dance with others. DMT is more than exercises, and it has become a language. It has the potential to improve psychological and emotional health by enhancing self-awareness and self-control and improving interpersonal function.

As psychiatrists, we are more concerned about how well DMT works with patients of mental disorders. According to the report of WHO [2], the global number of patients with depression increased by 18.4% every year from 2005 to 2015, and now there are more than 322 million patients. The number of people suffering from anxiety disorders is increasing by about 14.9% per year and now exceeds 260 million. Severe mental disorder schizophrenia is not as common as other mental disorders. It affects 20 million people worldwide and is associated with considerable disability.

J. Ren (✉) · C. Zhang
Shanghai Mental Health Center, Shanghai Jiaotong University School of Medicine, Shanghai, China

Shanghai Key Laboratory of Psychotic Disorders, Shanghai Mental Health Center, Shanghai Jiaotong University School of Medicine, Shanghai, China

C. Ye
Department of Psychological Medicine, Zhong Shan Hospital, Fudan University, Shanghai, China

U. Volpe (ed.), *Arts Therapies in Psychiatric Rehabilitation*,
https://doi.org/10.1007/978-3-030-76208-7_13

Till now, the most important treatment of mental disorders is medication. However, conventional medical treatments do not sufficiently address all symptoms and many can cause additional side effects. Researches in Taiwan found that the incidence of metabolic syndrome in patients with chronic schizophrenia is as high as 37.8% [3]. Metabolic problems are associated with a variety of factors, including diet habits, physical exercise, and the use of antipsychotic drugs [4]. It was found that although most patients with schizophrenia are very concerned about their weight and blood glucose, they are not willing to control metabolic problems by changing diet and increasing physical exercise [5]. Therefore, rehabilitation therapy plays an important role in alleviating symptoms, enabling patients to readapt to society, totally restoring their social functions, and keeping them fit as well [6].

It is obvious that there are developing trends about overall approach. However, its effectiveness must be tested in rigorous manner so as to provide a solid evidence for its use. Unfortunately, empirical evidence is sparse due to the small sample sizes and poor quality of studies. Moreover, the efficacy of DMT cannot really be addressed with studies of different types of dance; the abilities retained by different patients may vary greatly and unpredictably affect their cognitive functions and their ability to enjoy artistic experience [7].

Rigorous clinical researches have rarely been performed, with a few remarkable exceptions. Priebe et al. conducted a randomized controlled study, in which 275 schizophrenic patients were randomized into DMT and active group, respectively. Comprehensive outcomes including clinical effectiveness, satisfaction with treatment, adverse events, quality of life, social function, and cost were reported. These results showed that DMT does not have clinically meaningful benefits in the treatment of patients with negative symptoms of schizophrenia. However, the authors suggested that DMT may be a way to decrease social isolation and increase physical activity levels; it can be successfully implemented in the community for the high participant attendance [8].

Unlike traditional psychotherapy, DMT increases ability to create mind–body connections and improves physical health [9]. It can be used with people of all ages and practiced in various settings in the form of individual or group therapy. Overall, DMT has emerged as a promising alternative for patients with mental disorders. As stated in this chapter, it is important for DMT therapist to learn the "recovery language" and keep updated with current approaches in mental health so that they can better convey the advantages of using DMT for enhancing the integration of core recovery topics. On the other hand, we should bear in mind the chronicity and impact of mental disorder, and the most important outcomes would be real-world, patient-based meaningful outcomes. The rehabilitation road of patients of mental disorders should NOT be difficult and tough, but it is supposed to be a road full of hope and fun. Undoubtedly, DMT is among the most powerful methods to help the patients.

References

1. American Dance Therapy Association. What is dance/movement therapy? 2020. https://adta.org/clinical-info-sheets/.
2. Friedrich MJ. Depression is the leading cause of disability around the world. JAMA. 2017;317(15):1517.
3. Yang CY, Lo SC, Peng YC. Prevalence and predictors of metabolic syndrome in people with schizophrenia in inpatient rehabilitation wards. Biol Res Nurs. 2016;18(5):558–66.
4. Vancampfort D, Probst M, Scheewe T, De Herdt A, Sweers K, Knapen J, et al. Relationships between physical fitness, physical activity, smoking and metabolic and mental health parameters in people with schizophrenia. Psychiatry Res. 2013;207(1–2):25–32.
5. Sugawara N, Yasui-Furukori N, Yamazaki M, Shimoda K, Mori T, Sugai T, et al. Attitudes toward metabolic adverse events among patients with schizophrenia in Japan. Neuropsychiatr Dis Treat. 2016;12:427–36.
6. GBD 2017 Disease and Injury Incidence and Prevalence Collaborators. Global, regional, and national incidence, prevalence, and years lived with disability for 354 diseases and injuries for 195 countries and territories, 1990-2017: a systematic analysis for the Global Burden of Disease Study 2017. Lancet. 2018;392(10159):1789–858.
7. Mirabella G. Is art therapy a reliable tool for rehabilitating people suffering from brain/mental diseases? J Altern Complement Med. 2015;21(4):196–9.
8. Priebe S, Savill M, Wykes T, Bentall R, Lauber C, Reininghaus U, et al. Clinical effectiveness and cost-effectiveness of body psychotherapy in the treatment of negative symptoms of schizophrenia: a multicentre randomised controlled trial. Health Technol Assess. 2016;20(11):vii–xxiii, 1–100.
9. Levine B, Land HM. A meta-synthesis of qualitative findings about dance/movement therapy for individuals with trauma. Qual Health Res. 2016;26(3):330–44.

Neurophysiological Aspects of Dance Movement Therapy for Psychiatric Rehabilitation

14

Tal Shafir

Over the years, psychiatry has changed from having a psychotherapeutic (psychoanalytic) approach during the first half of the twentieth century to having mainly a biological, neuro-psychopharmacological approach during the end of the twentieth century and beginning of the twenty-first century [1]. In recent years, more and more voices are calling to integrate both of these approaches, either by treating with both types of therapy together [2] or by suggesting scientific models to the human mind, which integrate biological findings with psychological concepts, such as the neuropsychoanalysis approach [3]. The chapter by Wengrower and Bendel-Rozow relates to psychiatry primarily as a psychotherapeutic intervention and discusses how dance movement therapy (DMT) with psychiatric patients corresponds with this approach and approved to be effective. In my commentary, I will give examples to how the mechanisms underlying DMT methods and effects can be explained also by recent neuroscientific findings, making DMT an effective intervention also based on the biological and the integrative approaches to psychiatric rehabilitation.

According to peripheral theories of emotion, which were originated by Darwin and reformulated in neurophysiological terms by Damasio, emotions are generated by conveying the current state of the body to the brain [4]. This proposition implies that people can regulate their emotions by deliberately changing their motor behavior and its consequent proprioception and interoception. Indeed, many studies have shown that aerobic movement can affect the release of hormones, neurotransmitters, and neurotrophic factors in the brain and consequently, change one's emotional state and reduce the severity of psychiatric disorders such as stress, depression, and anxiety [5]. Other studies have shown that certain movement patterns are associated in the brain with specific emotions [6], probably through their unique proprioceptive input to the brain, and that moving these movement patterns can enhance the

T. Shafir (✉)
The Academic College for Society and Art, Netanya, Israel

The Emili Sagol Creative Arts Therapies Research Center, University of Haifa, Haifa, Israel
e-mail: tshafir1@univ.haifa.ac.il

U. Volpe (ed.), *Arts Therapies in Psychiatric Rehabilitation*,
https://doi.org/10.1007/978-3-030-76208-7_14

associated emotions [5–7]. Dance movement therapists encourage their clients to express, explore, and process their feelings through movement and lead their clients to regulate their emotions by suggesting to move with specific movement patterns, which enhance the associated desired emotions, and/or to reduce and avoid motor patterns associated with undesired emotions [8]. Thus, the effects of DMT in psychiatric rehabilitation can be explained also by their underlying neurophysiological emotion-regulation mechanisms, compatible with the biological approach.

Another neurophysiological finding underlying the methodology and effects of DMT is the mirror neurons. Mirror neurons are activated very similarly during motor execution and during motor observation of the same movements and are suggested to create in the observer's brain an internal simulation of the observed movements, leading to empathy [9] and elicitation of the same emotion as that felt by the mover [10]. Indeed, we found that observation of video clips of people expressing emotions through movements slightly enhanced the associated emotions in the observer [7]. Moreover, when people observed the same clips while their brain was scanned using functional magnetic resonance imaging (fMRI), observing movements that were associated with different emotions resulted with differential brain activation pattern (Fig. 14.1, personal data). In addition to significant activation in some brain regions (e.g., bilateral occipital cortex, bilateral inferior frontal gyrus/anterior insula, bilateral thalamus,) which was common to observing all types of emotional movements compared to observing non-emotional movements, only observing the happy movements significantly activated the ventral striatum, which has a role in reward and motivation; only observing fear movements significantly activated the parietal and motor cortex, probably as a preparation for fear-related actions (fight or flight), and only observing the sad movements resulted with reduced overall brain activation, consistent with the unresponsiveness and passivity (inactivity) that often accompany being sad. These findings support the idea of associations in the brain between certain movement patterns and specific emotions.

Dance movement therapists often mirror their client's movements, or join their movements in other ways. According to Koole and Tschacher's Interpersonal Synchrony model, movement synchrony should facilitate interbrain coupling, and this helps to establish alliance between the client and therapist, which in turn promotes adaptive emotion regulation in the patient, and thereby good therapeutic outcomes [11]. Although more research is needed to confirm this model, evidence supporting it are starting to accumulate [12]. This model, which integrates biological findings with psychological theory, can also explain the effectiveness of DMT in psychiatric rehabilitation.

Porges' Polyvagal Theory is a body–mind model which links the evolution of the mammalian autonomic nervous system to social behavior and emphasizes the importance of physiological state in the expression of behavioral problems and psychiatric disorders. DMT intervention principles conform with this theory as well, in particular in the treatment of trauma [13] and autism [14].

In summary, although DMT is a nonpharmacological intervention, its positive effects on mental health can be explained and understood not only using a

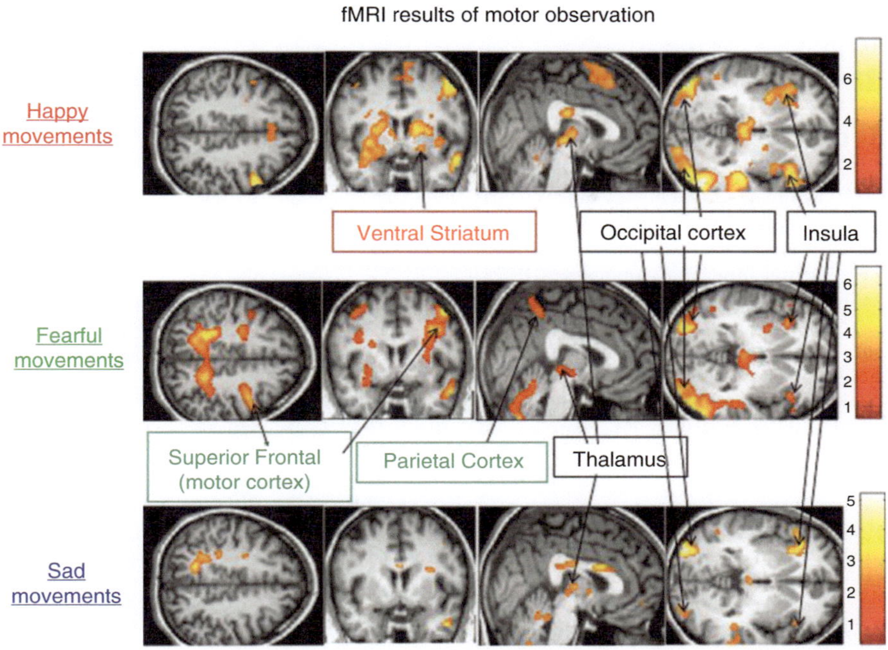

Fig. 14.1 Effects of observing happy, fearful and sad movements on brain activation. This figure shows brain activation during observation of emotional movements compared to observation of non-emotional movements. The top row of images includes four brain slices showing significant brain activation during observation of happy movements compared to observation of non-emotional movements. The middle row shows the same four slices during observation of fearful vs. non-emotional movements, and the lower row shows the same four brain slices during observation of sad compared to non-emotional movements. As can be seen, some regions (occipital cortex, insula, thalamus: all marked with black letters in a black box in the figure), whose activation relates to the general process of translating visual motor input into emotions, were activated during observation of all types of emotional movements and show significant activation in all three rows. In contrast, activation in other regions was specific to observing movements that express specific emotion: observation of only the happy movements created significant activation in the ventral striatum which is responsible for reward and motivation (upper row, marked in red letters); only observing fear movements significantly activated the parietal cortex (responsible for spatial orientation) and a much larger area in the motor cortex compared to that activated by observation of happy and sad movements. These regions were activated probably as part of preparation for *fight or flight* (second row, marked with green letters); observing the sad movements resulted with overall very low brain activation, consistent with the passivity and inactivity that often accompany being sad

psychotherapeutic approach to psychiatric rehabilitation but also from a neurophysiological perspective.

References

1. Reidbord S. A brief history of psychiatry: biology and psychology wrestle for the upper hand. Psychology Today.com; 2014.
2. Iannitelli A, et al. Psychodynamically oriented psychopharmacotherapy: towards a necessary synthesis. Front Hum Neurosci. 2019;13:15.
3. Panksepp J, Solms M. What is neuropsychoanalysis? Clinically relevant studies of the minded brain. Trends Cogn Sci. 2012;16(1):6–8.
4. Damasio A, Carvalho GB. The nature of feelings: evolutionary and neurobiological origins. Nat Rev Neurosci. 2013;14(2):143–52.
5. Shafir T. Movement-based strategies for emotion regulation. In: Bryant ML, editor. Handbook on emotion regulation: processes, cognitive effects and social consequences. New York: Nova Science; 2015. p. 231–49.
6. Shafir T, Tsachor RP, Welch KB. Emotion regulation through movement: unique sets of movement characteristics are associated with and enhance basic emotions. Front Psychol. 2016;6:2030.
7. Shafir T, et al. Emotion regulation through execution, observation, and imagery of emotional movements. Brain Cogn. 2013;82(2):219–27.
8. Tsachor RP, Shafir T. A somatic movement approach to fostering emotional resiliency through laban movement analysis. Front Hum Neurosci. 2017;11:410.
9. Decety J. Dissecting the neural mechanisms mediating empathy. Emot Rev. 2011;3(1):92–108.
10. Gallese V, Sinigaglia C. What is so special about embodied simulation? Trends Cogn Sci. 2011;15(11):512–9.
11. Koole SL, Tschacher W. Synchrony in psychotherapy: a review and an integrative framework for the therapeutic alliance. Front Psychol. 2016;7:862.
12. Zhang Y, et al. Interpersonal brain synchronization associated with working alliance during psychological counseling. Psychiatry Res Neuroimaging. 2018;282:103–9.
13. Dieterich-Hartwell R. Dance/movement therapy in the treatment of post traumatic stress: a reference model. Arts Psychother. 2017;54:38–46.
14. Devereaux C. Neuroception and attunement in dance/movement therapy with autism. Am J Dance Ther. 2017;39(1):36–8.

The Psychiatry-Related European DMT Experience

15

Vincenzo Puxeddu

Modern DMT has found its first application in the psychiatric field; experiences such as that of Marian Chace are an example. Experiences reverberated throughout Europe with other DMT pioneers such as Rose Gaertner, active since the 1950s, Santos Dumond Hospital in Paris; France Schott-Bilmann [1] also in France, in Greece and in Italy and Trudi Schoop in Switzerland. DMT then was developed by thousands of professionals throughout Europe up to the present day [2].

DMT has developed across the continent through the creation of National Professional Associations, which have been established across Europe and in particular in the UK (ADMPUK, 1982) France (SFDT, 1984), Germany (BTD, 1995), Greece (GATD, 1993) and Italy (APID, 1997). Some Eastern European countries joined DMT later than 1980s, one of the first being Hungary, HAMDT (1992). These first five countries met in Bologna in March 1997 and formed the steering group, for an international association, what then became the EADMT—European Association of Dance Movement Therapy (www.EADMT.com). EADMT assures and promotes the quality of dance movement therapy practice and training in Europe for the protection of clients, professionals and institutions. The EADMT aims to nurture mutual respect of diversity and to foster exchange and collaboration between member countries. As of October 2019, EADMT has 26 national member countries and around 2200 practitioners Europe-wide. The countries most highly represented are: Germany with 422 practitioners; Italy with 282; the United Kingdom with 270 and the Netherlands with 100.

Today the European Association of Dance Movement Therapy is the main platform through which the diversity of DMT practice in Europe finds its full expression. Europe, therefore, now has a single DMT voice, which allows for differences while sharing common goals. The psychiatric fields continues to represent a privileged area of the application of DMT in all European countries. A survey carried out by APID in 2006 revealed that around half of Italian DMT professionals operated in

V. Puxeddu (✉)
DMT Master Program, René Descartes–Paris University, Paris, France

U. Volpe (ed.), *Arts Therapies in Psychiatric Rehabilitation*,
https://doi.org/10.1007/978-3-030-76208-7_15

the public health service and, specifically, in the psychosocial and psychiatric spheres. Numerous experiments have been on-going since the 1990s in Italy, following the recommendations of the National Objective Project "Protection of Mental Health 1998–2000," which underlined the need for spaces and movement for the psychiatric patient. For example, one of these was a project, at the S.P.D.C. (Psychiatric Diagnosis and Treatment Service) in Cagliari, Sardinia [3]: 118 patients (58 females and 60 males), aged between 20 and 77 years, were taken care of, for a total of 245 attendances, over 12 months. The biweekly sessions saw the participation of a minimum of 3 up to a maximum of 10 patients in an integrated group (operators–patients) for a total of 8–18 participants. The patients who participated were affected by various pathologies such as schizophrenia, bipolar disorder, depression, personality disorders and Neurosis. The evaluation of the project, aimed at improving the daily quality of life of patients hospitalized in the acute phase, took place on the basis of observation charts for movement and participation, and self-assessment questionnaires to be completed by patients and operators.

The study showed greater patient compliance with care activities, an improved patient–operator relationship, thanks to group experience. In general, a better quality of life is reported in the healthcare setting, on the basis of an investment in the space of the hospital department, in patient movement and socialisation terms.

The previous chapter provides us a broad view of the various elements of DMT at the base of this practice, thus linked to psychosocial rehabilitation, which in Italy has seen a multiplication of experiences [4], through multiple approaches to DMT.

DMT has its origins in the history of humanity itself, the therapeutic dance rituals mentioned in the previous chapter, the figure of the shaman at the base of the practice of dance and art, but it also is a reference to the care of the individual and of the community, and all these have found in ethno-psychiatry a psychoanalytic reinterpretation of treatment activity. Among these we have mentioned the contribution of ethno-psychiatry in France in the psychoanalytic rereading of possession rituals and, in general, of therapeutic dance rituals. From this root comes the contemporary anthropological approach to DMT, which enriches this practice with technical and theoretical elements, enhancing the contribution of rhythm, the group, the ground and the ritual. I would like to report a preliminary study carried out at Athens University Psychiatric Clinic in Greece [5], which concerns a specific dance therapy technique, called primitive expression (PE), providing physical and neuropsychological benefits. It involves ethnologically and socially based forms, which are supplied for re-enactment, as well as an incentive for successful performance. In PE, play, rhythm, dance and song work together at a symbolic level. The aim is to encourage participants to act and express themselves, while orienting their drives in a positive way. This chapter presents preliminary results of a PE-based protocol with a small group of 11 psychiatric patients, with psychotic and depressive disorders. It is shown that a relatively short duration of 12 PE sessions, twice a week, for 6 weeks of treatment, led to observable changes in psychological state, behaviour and brain physiology. It was found that the patients experienced an increase in their happiness level (OHQ—Oxford Happiness Questionnaire), expressed a positive attitude to the PE process by using appropriate word associations (WAQ—Word

Association Questionnaire) and exhibited (in a patient subset) an increase in EEG activity related to a relaxed waking state. This study presents encouraging results relating to the application of PE therapy in psychiatric patients. PE can be added to other dance therapy methodologies which have been shown to be promising therapeutic approaches in psychiatric populations.

In conclusion, there are many experiences in Europe characterized by the presence of DMT, both in rehabilitative settings, such as day hospitals, and in psychiatric services. In general, its positive effect on patients' bodily, communication and relational skills is much appreciated. DMT is identified as a complementary activity, in pursuing care goals, and is effective also in the mitigation reactions characterized by maladaptation.

References

1. Schott-Bilmann France. Quand la danse guérit. Paris: Coll.La recherche en danse; 1994.
2. Puxeddu V. La Danse Therapie, Les Art-Therapies, a cura di Lecourt E. e Loubart T. Malakoff (France): Armand Colin – Dounod Editore; 2017, p. 120–155.
3. Puxeddu V, Baraldi A, Camerada V, Lilliu F, Pili P, Turri P, Zedda MV. Psichiatria e DanzaMovimentoTerapia Integrata®- un'esperienza presso il Servizio di Diagnosi e Cura dell'Ospedale is Mirrionis di Cagliari. DanzaMovimentoTerapia - Modelli e pratiche nell'esperienza Italiana, / ed. Apid, a cura di Adorisio A, Garcia ME, Roma: Edizioni MAGI; 2004.p. 195–216.
4. Ba G. Strumenti e tecniche di riabilitazione psichiatrica e psicosociale, Franco Angeli; 2004.
5. Margariti A, Ktonas P, Hondraki P, Daskalopoulou E, Kyriakopoulos G, Economou NT, Tsekou H, Paparrigopoulos T, Barbousi V, Vaslamatzis G. An application of the primitive expression form of dance therapy in a psychiatric population. Arts Psychother. 2012;39:95–101.

Listening to the Voice of the Person with Psychiatric Problems

16

Rosa-María Rodríguez-Jiménez

In the search for evidence in arts-based interventions within the field of psychiatry, there are several concepts to consider—as Wengrower and Bendel-Rozow do: the psychiatric rehabilitation model itself, the idiosyncrasy of the therapeutic approach, in this case dance movement therapy (DMT), and finally, the research and evidence-based contributions, to which it would be appropriate to add a review of the paradigm itself.

In recent years, the treatment of severe mental illness has been moving towards so-called functional recovery. While there are different interpretations of what "recovery" actually means, there is a shared basis that refers to enabling people with psychiatric problems to achieve their personal goals. The World Psychiatric Association highlighted that "the aim of psychosocial rehabilitation is to support people with severe mental illness in developing their cognitive, emotional and social skills, in order to live in the community with the slightest professional sustenance." The concept of psychosocial rehabilitation is oriented to work on the strengths and capacities that each patient has, regardless of their clinical condition [1]. Authors such as Frost et al. [2] also propose a model based on the person's own needs: improved functioning and the sense of hope and possibility and increased skills and reconnection with the community. Davidson et al. [3] had previously expanded the concept of recovery, to talk about inclusion, acceptance of difference, and "simply to be let in" based on three areas: (a) social inclusion, (b) feeling like a worthwhile human being, and (c) hopefulness. They also insisted on the need to review our current models of mental illness and its treatment.

Art therapies, and in particular DMT, share many of these objectives by offering a nondirective work environment—of listening to the person in the here and now (empathic resonance). This approach offers a response to the intervention proposals with positive results in the reduction of negative symptoms, self-knowledge,

R.-M. Rodríguez-Jiménez (✉)
Universidad Europea de Madrid, Madrid, Spain
e-mail: rosamaria.rodriguez@universidadeuropea.es

U. Volpe (ed.), *Arts Therapies in Psychiatric Rehabilitation*,
https://doi.org/10.1007/978-3-030-76208-7_16

awareness, and relational skills [1, 4]. At the same time, DMT is integrated into the clinical service in many countries, but due to its cross-sectoral nature [5], it is used in social and/or educational contexts and in prevention [6] outside the traditional hospital environment. This has a special interest for a population that, due to its affectation, has difficulties in its inclusion in social life.

As developed in the main chapter, the fundamental principles of DMT are the conception of embodiment, the body awareness, the meaning of symbolic movement, and the creative process in a context of therapeutic alliance. The term embodiment [7] has been widely studied in the last decades since neuroscience [8, 9] revealed that cognitive structures are formed from a physical body and that there is a continuous relationship of communication and learning between different body structures (including mental structures) and biological mechanisms. DMT works with the relationship between movement and emotional response, knowing that changes in the form and qualities of movement also produce changes at the physiological level [10, 11]. In addition, the particularity of working with the symbolic meaning of the nonverbal in a transitional space [12] generates the development of the creative and indistinct expression of each individual [13].

The last concept dealt with refers to evidence from DMT. As mentioned by Wrengower and Bendel-Rozow, studies on DMT interventions according to the evidence-based practice (EBP) paradigm have increased in recent years, although they remain scarce. EBP brought in from the clinical field is characterized by a set of criteria to guarantee that all interventions are effective based on rigorous research. In this context, one research methodology—the randomized controlled trial (RCT)—is preferred above all others [14]. Collected studies/reviews of DMT in depression [15–17], schizophrenia [18], and dementia [11, 19], for instance, show the difficulties in meeting Cochrane's strict criteria, such as limited sample sizes or different treatment approaches, despite their important contribution to clinical work with different populations. Slade et al. [20] underlined that "evidence-based mental healthcare" does not mean "RCT-based mental healthcare." Organizations such as the National Institute for Health Research or the Campbell Collaboration believe that qualitative and process-oriented approaches generate knowledge in the advancement of best clinical practice and must be considered. They allow a better understanding of mental problems along with contextual and cultural factors, and more importantly, they include the voice of the person with a mental issue. Authors such as O'Cathain et al. [21] and Strassel et al. [22] highlight the contribution of mixed methods in the field of mental health. In fact, the introduction of mixed methodologies for studying the effects of DMT interventions has increased significantly in recent years for different mental illnesses [23–25]. The recovery-oriented dance movement therapy (RODMT) presented in the chapter is a good example of the mixed approach for recovery proposals [26].

Gilbody and Sowden [27] suggest that professions should first identify what is the definition of evidence and establish what makes this profession unique, prior to looking for significant research questions and how to answer them. This means defining their own evidential standards and the appropriate levels of evidence, such that the research methods are put to the service of answering research questions, and not the reverse [28]. In fact, the same meta-analysis [13] mentioned in the chapter incorporates only controlled studies, but connects the results to the intervention characteristics. EBP in psychological therapies comes directly from clinical work, and so observations should be systematically documented and described through case studies or other appropriate methods [29]. Gilroy [14] suggests to construct a hierarchy of levels and include together with the RCTs research methods that come from the arts and social sciences, such as case studies, phenomenological, ethnographic, anthropological, and art-based and collaborative studies [30, 31]. To this end, it is necessary to establish guidelines that structure the evidence of the interventions with criteria of validity and applicability [32]. This would provide greater adjustment to EBP by reconciling quantitative outcomes of the interventions with the processes that give more space to what patients say about their own experiences. Going back to Gilroy's words, adapted to the DMT field: "we need the facts, we need the figures, but we need the stories and the [dances] too."

References

1. Vita A, Barlati S. The implementation of evidence-based psychiatric rehabilitation: challenges and opportunities for mental health services. Front Psychiatry. 2019;10(MAR):1–5. https://doi.org/10.3389/fpsyt.2019.00147.
2. Frost BG, Tirupati S, Johnston S, Turrell M, Lewin TJ, Sly KA, Conrad AM. An Integrated Recovery-oriented Model (IRM) for mental health services: evolution and challenges. BMC Psychiatry. 2017;17(1):1–17. https://doi.org/10.1186/s12888-016-1164-3.
3. Davidson L, Stayner DA, Nickou C, Styron TH, Rowe M, Chinman ML. 'Simply to be let in': inclusion as a basis for recovery. Psychiatr Rehabil J. 2001;24:375–88. https://doi.org/10.1037/h0095067.
4. Stuckey HL, Nobel J. The connection between art, healing, and public health: a review of current literature. Am J Public Health. 2010;100(2):254–63. https://doi.org/10.2105/AJPH.2008.156497.
5. Barry M, Clarke A, Petersen I, Jenkins R. Implementing mental health promotion. Basel: Springer Nature; 2019.
6. Payne H. The body speaks its mind: the BodyMind Approach® for patients with medically unexplained symptoms in primary care in England. Arts Psychother. 2015;42:19–27. https://doi.org/10.1016/j.aip.2014.12.011.
7. Koch S, Fuchs T. Embodied arts therapies. Arts Psychother. 2011;38:276–80. https://doi.org/10.1016/j.aip.2011.08.007.
8. Damasio A. The feeling of what happens: body and emotion in the making of consciousness. London: Harcourt Inc.; 1999.
9. Damasio A. Self comes to mind: constructing the conscious brain. New York, NY: Pantheon; 2012.
10. Jeong YJ, Hong SC, Myeong SL, Park MC, Kim YK, Suh CM. Dance movement therapy improves emotional responses and modulates neurohormones in adolescents with mild depression. Int J Neurosci. 2005;115(12):1711–20. https://doi.org/10.1080/00207450590958574.
11. Koch S, Kunz T, Lykou S, Cruz R. Effects of dance movement therapy and dance on health-related psychological outcomes: a meta-analysis. Arts Psychother. 2014;41(1):46–64. https://doi.org/10.1016/j.aip.2013.10.004.
12. Winnicott DW. Playing and reality. London: Tavistock Publications; 1971.

13. Koch SC, Riege RFF, Tisborn K, Biondo J, Martin L, Beelmann A. Effects of dance movement therapy and dance on health-related psychological outcomes. A meta-analysis update. Front Psychol. 2019;10(AUG):1806. https://doi.org/10.3389/fpsyg.2019.01806.
14. Gilroy A. Art therapy, research and evidence-based practice. London: Sage Publications, Inc.; 2006.
15. Jiménez J, Bräuninger I, Meekums B. Dance movement therapy with older people with a psychiatric condition: a systematic review. Arts Psychother. 2019;63:118–27. https://doi.org/10.1016/j.aip.2018.11.008.
16. Karkou V, Aithal S, Zubala A, Meekums B. Effectiveness of dance movement therapy in the treatment of adults with depression: a systematic review with meta-analyses. Front Psychol. 2019;10(APR):936. https://doi.org/10.3389/fpsyg.2019.00936.
17. Pylvänäinen PM, Muotka JS, Lappalainen R. A dance movement therapy group for depressed adult patients in a psychiatric outpatient clinic: effects of the treatment. Front Psychol. 2015;6(July):1–11. https://doi.org/10.3389/fpsyg.2015.00980.
18. Ren J, Xia J. Dance therapy for schizophrenia. Cochrane Database Syst Rev. 2013;10:CD006868. https://doi.org/10.1002/14651858.CD006868.pub3.
19. Lyons S, Karkou V, Roe B, Meekums B, Richards M. What research evidence is there that dance movement therapy improves the health and wellbeing of older adults with dementia? A systematic review and descriptive narrative summary. Arts Psychother. 2018;60:32–40. https://doi.org/10.1016/j.aip.2018.03.006.
20. Slade M, Kuipers E, Priebe S. Mental health services research methodology. Int Rev Psychiatry. 2002;14:12. https://doi.org/10.1080/09540260120114014.
21. O'Cathain A, Thomas KJ, Drabble SJ, Rudolph A, Goode J, Hewison J. Maximising the value of combining qualitative research and randomised controlled trials in health research: the QUAlitative Research in Trials (QUART) study - a mixed methods study. Health Technol Assess. 2014;18(38):1–197. https://doi.org/10.3310/hta18380.
22. Strassel JK, Cherkin DC, Steuten L, Sherman KJ, Vrijhoef M, Hubertus J. A systematic review of the evidence for the effectiveness of dance therapy. Altern Ther Health Med. 2011;17(3):50–9.
23. Bryl K. The role of dance/movement therapy in the treatment of negative syndrome and psychosocial functioning of patients with schizophrenia: result from a pilot mixed methods intervention study with explanatory intent. Schizophr Bull. 2018;44(1):315–6. https://www.ncbi.nlm.nih.gov/pmc/articles/PMC5887448/.
24. Coaten ME. Dance Movement Psychotherapy (DMP) in acute adult. 2020. http://etheses.dur.ac.uk/13548/.
25. Savidaki M, Demirtoka S, Rodríguez-Jiménez R-M. Re-inhabiting one's body: a pilot study on the effects of dance movement therapy on body image and alexithymia in eating disorders. J Eat Disord. 2020;8(1):1–20. https://doi.org/10.1186/s40337-020-00296-2.
26. Bendel-Rozow T. Recovery-oriented dance movement therapy: a controlled trial in mental health rehabilitation. Expressive Therapies Dissertations. 2020. https://digitalcommons.lesley.edu/expressive_dissertations/98.
27. Gilbody S, Sowden A. Systematic reviews in mental health. In: Rowland N, Goss S, editors. Evidence-based counselling and psychological therapies: research and applications. London: Routledge; 2000. p. 216.
28. Rodríguez-Jiménez R-M, Carmona M. Mixed methods for evaluating embodied processes in higher education. In: Tantia J, editor. The art and science of embodied research design: concepts, methods and cases. New York, NY: Routledge Press; 2020.
29. Roth A, Fonagy P. What works for whom? A critical review of psychotherapy research. New York, NY: Guildford; 1996.
30. Eberhard-Kaechele M. A political perspective on dance movement psychotherapy on interdisciplinary pathways: are we finding or losing our way?*. Body Move Dance Psychother. 2017;12(4):237–51. https://doi.org/10.1080/17432979.2017.1372521.

31. Hanvey C, Tepper-Lewis C. Co-leading for community building: a program description of a dual-modality creative arts therapy group in psychiatric emergency care. Arts Psychother. 2019;66:101581. https://doi.org/10.1016/j.aip.2019.101581.
32. Fenner P, Abdelazim RS, Bräuninger I, Strehlow G, Seifert K. Provision of arts therapies for people with severe mental illness. Curr Opin Psychiatry. 2017;30(4):306–11. https://doi.org/10.1097/YCO.0000000000000338.

Part IV

Drama Theatre Therapy

Drama Therapy in the Context of Psychiatric Care

17

Nisha Sajnani

17.1 Introduction

Throughout human history, drama and theatre have allowed human beings to move from the *as-is* to the *as-if*, the realm of make-believe. In dramatic reality, we are afforded the opportunity to temporarily suspend the plausible in order to explore the possible. Drama therapy, a term that is used interchangeably with theatre therapy, allows one to experience, in the present, events that have occurred in the past or that may occur in the future, try out new roles, rehearse adaptive verbal and nonverbal responses to challenging situations, practice navigating the line between the real and the imagined, and reinforce spontaneity and creativity. For these and other reasons, drama therapy is a suitable approach for use in psychiatric contexts. This chapter provides a brief overview of the history of drama therapy, primary techniques and available evidence in the context of psychiatric rehabilitation, and recommendations for future directions.

17.2 History

The use of dramatic processes to promote well-being and alleviate distressing symptoms in individuals and communities can be traced back to indigenous, mystic, and spiritual healing rituals in early Africa, China, Egypt, India, Persia, then later in Greece and Italy [1–7]. Early healers intuited that to treat the sick, one had to engage directly with the patient, not only with prescriptive words and therapeutic touch but also with expressive forms of movement, sound, word, mask, and image-making in order to make contact with the spirit world that exists in the imaginal realm, both

N. Sajnani (✉)
Program in Drama Therapy and the Theatre and Health Lab, New York University, New York, NY, USA
e-mail: nisha.sajnani@nyu.edu

U. Volpe (ed.), *Arts Therapies in Psychiatric Rehabilitation*,
https://doi.org/10.1007/978-3-030-76208-7_17

within and beyond the body [6, 8]. Early written documentations such as Bharatmuni's Natyashastra (circa 500–300 BC), the Indian treatise on dance, music, and drama, and Aristotle's Poetics (335 BC, [9]), its Greek counterpart, asserted the value of dramatic imitation in arousing and immersing audiences in an illusion intended to inspire wonder, contemplation, and reinforce moral ideals [10, 11]. Aristotle's singular use of the word "catharsis" to connote the purging of emotions of pity and fear when one watches a tragedy is often referenced as an early example of the psychological and social benefits of drama and theatre. Through a process of recognizing the limits of one's power, as is often the case in a tragedy, the spectator is thought to be brought to a greater sense of self-knowledge and a commitment to prevailing, though not necessarily ideal, social norms.

Moving towards contemporary practice, several innovations unfolded in the fields of psychology, sociology, anthropology, and theatre between the late eighteenth and early twentieth century that converged to lay the groundwork for the contemporary practice of drama therapy. This section will touch on just a few. Innovations took place in hospitals wherein patients would engage in theatrical performances in psychiatric and rehabilitation facilities in England, Germany, France, Italy, Poland, Hungary, Austria, and Russia [3]. Carl Jung, Otto Rank, Sandor Ferenczi, and Wilhelm Reich, while upholding the importance of Freud's study of the psyche, each challenged his overreliance on logical analysis, which they viewed as a rational means toward uncovering an irrational psychological structure, and advocated the benefits of working holistically through visual images, stories, physical enactments, and active engagement with patients [8]. The developments of these early pioneers led to the action-oriented innovations by J.L. Moreno, Fritz Perls, and Virginia Satir among others.

J.L. Moreno, an Austrian psychiatrist, began to experiment with action methods in Vienna in the 1920s. This led to the development of the *Stegreiftheater* (the "theatre of spontaneity"), where actors improvised scenes based on themes suggested by Moreno and the audience. Actors would also improvise and perform scenes based upon current events which Moreno referred to as *Living Newspaper* and used it as a forum to debate important issues. These early experiments by J.L. Moreno and his wife, Zerka, were organized into various approaches such as *sociometry*, *sociodrama*, *monodrama*, and *psychodrama* and deeply influenced the group psychotherapy movement [12]. In Moreno's theatre, patients were invited to see their intra and interpersonal conflicts, as well as their symptoms externalized on stage. By role-playing their psychological world, Moreno asserted that patients could develop their "observing ego" which distanced them from their emotions and permitted a greater degree of insight and self-control [13]. Moreno's innovations brought into existence a comprehensive approach to the use of action methods in psychotherapy.

Meanwhile, theatre theorists and practitioners began to experiment and amplify the psychological properties of acting, the ability to "live truthfully under imaginary circumstances" ([14], p. 15). The most significant of these included Konstantin Stanislavski who stressed the relationship between authentic affective experiencing and physical action in contrast to acting as representation alone [15]; Bertholt

Brecht who emphasized the value of theatrical distancing in facilitating critical thinking; Jerzy Grotowski who focused attention on psychophysical action and the primacy of the encounter between actor and audience; Augusto Boal [16] whose *Theatre of the Oppressed* invited groups to act collectively to challenge and seek out solutions to prevailing sociocultural norms which, from his perspective, led to psychological distress; and Viola Spolin who illuminated the social benefits of improvisation [17]. It is in the convergence of artistic, and psychotherapeutic experiments with imagination, action, and role and theatrical explorations of psychological and social truths, that drama therapy emerged as a profession.

17.2.1 The Emergence of Drama Therapy

The first documented use of the term "drama therapy" was in 1917 wherein dramatic performance was valued for its vitalizing effects on the performer and the audience [18, 19]. However, the profession of drama therapy is often attributed to two major trends in the United Kingdom and the United States. In the UK, Peter Slade first used the term *dramatherapy* (spelled as one word in the UK) in his 1939 address to the British Medical Association about the value of drama in the treatment of children with disabilities and behavioral difficulties [20]. Sue Jennings began to develop remedial drama for use with differently abled populations; over 40 years of practice, she defined key concepts and provided clear technical descriptions of the intentional use of drama to promote health and well-being with a wide variety of populations across the lifespan [21–25]. Marian Lindkvist also pioneered the early profession of drama therapy in the UK, opening up a center of drama and movement called Sesame and training generations of practitioners [26]. Jennings and Lindquist were followed by important practitioners and thinkers such as Alida Gersie [27] who advanced our understanding of the use of stories and storytelling in therapy and Phil Jones [4] who first articulated core therapeutic processes in drama therapy. In the United States, the field of drama therapy was pioneered by a number of practitioners including actress and early pioneer of healing arts, Gertrude Schattner and educational theatre specialist Richard Courtney [28]; child psychoanalyst, Eleanor Irwin [17]; clinical psychologist, David Read Johnson who developed an ontological theory based in improvisational play [17]; Sesame-trained drama therapist, Renée Emunah who articulated an integrated "five-phase model" of drama therapy [29]; and theatre-trained Robert Landy who articulated a theory of personality and health involving the development and expansion of one's role repertoire [30, 31]. Johnson and Emunah [17], in their book entitled "Current Approaches in Drama Therapy," include descriptions of 22 different approaches that have been developed and/or used by American drama therapists from diverse theatrical and psychological orientations.

Drama therapy has since become embedded in graduate-level clinical training programs and is a recognized profession in over 30 countries. Drama therapists are trained in both the theory and practice of several psychotherapeutic, theatrical, and drama therapy approaches and are able to meet the academic, clinical, and ethical standards set by their professional associations ([32], www.worldallianceofdrama-therapy.com). While definitions across professional associations differ slightly, the distinguishing consistent feature of drama therapy is that it is an aesthetic therapy that makes use of fictional or "dramatic reality" [33] to give people a chance to work through past, present, and anticipated challenges with a greater degree of psychological or "aesthetic distance" [30].

Drama therapists attempt to consciously extend our natural capacities for play toward the realization of specific therapeutic goals with individuals and groups in the context of private practice, psychiatric and rehabilitation facilities, schools, elder care homes, prisons, and community centers. Participants in drama therapy work through play and their imaginative capacities to create roles and to tell, enact, and reflect upon their stories. Drama therapists work in partnership with participants and clinical teams to determine therapeutic goals, culturally and developmentally suitable ways of working, and to monitor and evaluate progress. The primary goal of drama therapeutic process is often to provide people with a safe and secure experience that facilitates emotional stability and creative expression through playful, dramatic activity and to address specific therapeutic objectives [34]. These may include the promotion of positive cognitive and behavioral changes, increased self-awareness, perspective-taking, and problem-solving, improved interpersonal relationship skills, enhanced emotional expression and modulation, fun, and pleasure, and improved overall quality of life.

17.3 Basic Principles and Techniques

In the context of psychiatry, drama therapists tend to work in four main areas: brief acute inpatient care, long-term inpatient care, outpatient care, and staff development [35–39]. A session of drama therapy typically involves a "warm up" phase to elicit salient themes, an action phase in which central themes are given focus through projective play, storymaking, and/or enactment, followed by a period of processing to facilitate the integration of material explored through drama, and closure. However, techniques may also be embedded within traditional talk psychotherapy. For example, *dramatic projection* techniques, in which inner feelings, fears, and wishes are concretized within a fictionalized role or inanimate object such as a figurine, mask, puppet, or text, are particularly useful in externalizing unconscious processes and clarifying issues and concerns. While objectives and techniques will vary depending on context, time, diagnosis, and clinical orientation, the following considerations and approaches have been documented in psychiatric settings.

In the context of acute care, drama therapeutic objectives tend to meet specific, stability-oriented goals while still promoting creativity, expression, and the benefits of working in a supportive relationship. Forrester and Johnson [40] point to the potential of *developmental transformations* (DvT), an approach that involves embodied, improvisational, relational play in drama therapy, in promoting optimism and active engagement in treatment to counter the demoralization, shame, isolation, and fear that those in brief inpatient care may experience. Reynolds [41] observed the value of this approach in aiding children in inpatient psychiatric contexts to "playfully represent anger" in a supportive therapeutic relationship (p. 299).

Ron [42] documented the role of psychodramatic techniques in alleviating acute distress in an open therapy group in inpatient psychiatry. In particular, he points to *mirroring* where the participant, referred to as the protagonist, works with the guidance of the therapist to enact a challenging experience and then step out of the scene to watch as another group member steps into their role and portrays them in the scene. In this case, group members become "auxiliary egos" allowing the protagonist to gain perspective on their experience. He also highlighted the value of the *role-playing*, where the protagonist takes on the role of themselves or others in their lives, and the *substituting role technique*, where the protagonist is invited to take on symbolic roles that are very different from themselves. In addition to these examples, the psychodramatic technique of *doubling*, where the therapist or other group members empathically verbalize thoughts or feelings that a protagonist may be unable to express during an enactment, is useful in individual or group work. The person being doubled may welcome or correct statements as necessary. *Role-reversal* is also useful in that it invites participants to empathize with the perspective of another and to see themselves through the other's eyes. Finally, the use of the *empty chair* technique is particularly potent in that it offers participants an opportunity to engage in a conversation with aspects of themselves or with individuals with whom they have unresolved concerns. This approach may be integrated with other techniques described above to facilitate aesthetic distance, an oscillation between emotional arousal and cognitive processing.

In long-term rehabilitation, greater consideration may be given to developing and addressing group themes and working through the source of specific symptoms, maladaptive schemas, and behaviors. Butler [43] observed the potential for DvT to alleviate negative symptoms of psychosis and expand flexibility in his work with people suffering from schizophrenia. Long-term care also presents opportunities to develop *therapeutic theatre* with groups if indicated. In this technique, individuals or groups work with a preexisting script that reflects themes of concerns to the group or devise original scenes that are then presented to a chosen audience, often consisting of family, care providers, and medical staff. The group that becomes a theatre ensemble, the script, and the audience each offer interpersonal structures that aid in organizing experience at increasing levels of distance through which participants may express themselves. Emunah and Johnson [44] observed the following benefits and challenges of this technique for the psychiatric patient:

> Tremendous pressures are mobilized internally and externally for changes in self-image. The risks involved are contained by the support of the group and the drama therapist who is responsible for monitoring the impact of the experience. The intensity of this impact seems to be particularly affected by … the degree of the audience's awareness of the patient status, … the degree to which the script reveals the personal lives of the patients, … [and] the degree to which the cast processes their personal relationships with each other and with their roles during the rehearsal period. (p. 239)

In outpatient care, documented therapeutic objectives include increasing social interaction, facilitating the release and control of emotions, changing nonconstructive behavioral and role patterns, developing imagination, spontaneity, and imagination, and increasing self-esteem and self-confidence [36]. Sajnani et al. [45] emphasized the use of *metaphor* in aiding participants suffering from depression to develop a coherent narrative about their experience; *dramatic projection*, where depression could be given form through different colored fabrics and objects; *dramatic embodiment*, where participants could create still sculptures using their bodies to convey a theme; *play* to instill a sense of spontaneity, recover laughter, and encourage a range of approaches to express inner experience; and *role-play* to support participants in embodying a dialogue between different and conflicting parts of themselves. Working through *role dissonance*, a core feature of the role method of drama therapy in psychiatric contexts, was also observed by Landy [30] and McMullian and Burch [46]. McAdam and Johnson [47] reported a decrease in depressive symptoms among adolescents suffering from posttraumatic stress disorder who participated in DvT. Clinical results reported by Pitre et al. [48] revealed the value of DvT as a means of facilitating gradual exposure and desensitization to triggering reminders of traumatic events.

The use of performance in psychiatric contexts is also a useful approach to supporting participants who are transitioning from a higher level of care as it can offer participants a structured group environment, a sense of purpose, and an opportunity to be seen by audiences in a role other than patient thereby disrupting stereotypes about mental illness [38]. Finally, with regard to staff development, drama therapeutic techniques may be used to help staff identify and represent feelings concerning challenging patients, rehearse responses to problems present in the organizational structure, examine the relationship between social factors and the presentation of psychological distress, and develop an increased sense of spontaneity and creativity [37].

17.4 Available Evidence

Research on drama therapy in the treatment of various psychiatric conditions yield promising results while pointing to the need for further research. In a Cochrane review of drama therapy in the treatment of schizophrenia and schizophrenia-like illnesses, Ruddy and Dent-Brown [49] noted the value of drama as an organizing scaffold for disordered thoughts and feelings; however, the results of the review were inconclusive due to poor reporting in the studies surveyed. Case examples from Casson [50], Butler [43], and Johnson [51, 52] with the same population reveal the value of drama therapy in representing internal experience and promoting change without insisting that participants be able to communicate insights. Crawford and Patterson [53], in their systematic review of the creative arts therapies in the treatment of schizophrenia, highlighted the emerging evidence that the arts therapies, including drama therapy, have a greater impact on negative symptoms such as withdrawal and reduced motivation than positive symptoms of psychosis. Ron [42] also documented an observable decrease in loneliness and distress for patients with various symptoms who participated in an open psychodrama group in an inpatient unit. Recent case evidence from Bielańska [13], whose implementation of five sessions of psychodrama spread over 10 weeks coupled with psychopharmacological treatment, resulted in an observable decrease in auditory hallucinations. A study of global assessment of functioning by Sancar et al. [54] of patients with severe mental illness revealed that drama therapy (1× week, 90 min sessions, ×24 weeks) resulted in a significant decrease in loss of functioning and high group means for hope, group cohesion, and altruism.

A randomized control trial conducted by Anari et al. [55] indicated that children who received drama therapy (2× week ×6 weeks) reported a significant decrease in symptoms of social anxiety disorder. A case study of the use of role method in the treatment of a woman with a documented personality disorder and anxiety revealed that drama therapy offered a sense of relief and control [56]. Moran and Alon [57] examined the effects of a 10-week (2× week, 75-min sessions) *playback theatre* protocol, a technique involving storytelling, enactment, and empathic listening on self-esteem, personal growth, and recovery of 19 adults with mental health disorders including schizophrenia, bipolar disorder, posttraumatic stress disorder, or chronic clinical depression. Results indicated enhanced self-esteem, self-knowledge, fun and relaxation, and an enhanced sense of connection and empathy for others. A systematic review on the use of the arts therapies in the treatment of depression among older adults revealed [58] that the opportunities for playful interaction and externalization of significant experiences that are characteristic of drama therapy reinforced internal resources and contributed to a sense of generativity among those participating in an average of 12 sessions.

In the context of forensic psychiatry, a pilot study by Keulen-de Vos et al. [59] with patients with cluster B personality disorders in a forensic psychiatry unit revealed that a five-session drama therapy protocol (1× week) based on Emunah's [29] five-phase model was effective in inducing vulnerable emotional states. This was also observed by Smeijsters and Cleven [60], whose qualitative study of the protocols and effects observed by 31 arts therapists across 12 institutions in the Netherlands and Germany indicated that drama therapy, along with other arts therapies, was instrumental in reducing recidivism among patients. Finally, studies by Orkibi et al. [61] and Yotis et al. [62] highlighted the value of drama therapy in decreasing the stigma associated with mental illness.

17.5 Future Directions

The present chapter provides an overview of the role of drama and theatre as therapy. Drama therapy has been used to help individuals and communities to express feelings, promote recovery, and improve overall well-being. It encourages flexibility, spontaneity, creativity, and collaboration which, as the case material and evidence suggests, is useful in managing anxiety, emotional regulation, and increasing a sense of personal and collective empowerment. While the available evidence is promising, further studies are needed to identify the therapeutic mechanisms particular to drama therapy and establish treatment guidelines for specific conditions. Mixed method approaches combining systematic, randomized controlled studies together with qualitative accounts that elevate the voices of those who participate in drama therapy are necessary. Publishing drama therapy treatment and research protocols, consistent and transparent reporting, the inclusion of social factors and nuanced demographic data, together with improvements in methodology would aid in determining the benefits and contraindications for the use of drama therapy in psychiatric contexts. Furthermore, it is imperative that future research consider not only implications for practice but also for policy as better data will facilitate increased access to this generative approach to care. Changing attitudes in psychiatry towards a greater degree of partnership in the context of care blend well with approaches in drama therapy that uniformly stress the importance of co-creation. Drama therapy has a promising future in the context of psychiatric rehabilitation.

References

1. Bailey MS, de Silva HJ. Sri Lankan sanni masks: an ancient classification of disease. BMJ. 2006;333:1327–8.
2. Brockett O, Hildy F. History of the theatre. Boston, MA: Allyn & Bacon; 2003.
3. Casson J. Dramatherapy history in headlines: who did what, when, where? Dramatherapy. 1997;19:10–3.
4. Jones P. Drama as therapy: theatre as living. London: Routledge; 1996.
5. Lewis P. Creative transformation: the healing power of the arts. Wilmette, IL: Chiron Publications; 1993.
6. Pendzik S. Drama therapy as a form of modern shamanism. Journal of Transpersonal Psychology. 1988;20:81–92.
7. Snow S. Ritual/theater/therapy. In: Johnson DR, Emunah R, editors. Current approaches in drama therapy. Springfield, IL: Charles C. Thomas; 2009. p. 117–44.
8. Landy R. The couch and the stage: integrating words and action in psychotherapy. New York, NY: The Rowman & Littlefield Publishing Group; 2008.
9. Aristotle. Poetics, I. Bywater, translator. New York, NY: Modern Library; 335 BC/1954.
10. Hartigan K. Performance and cure: drama and healing in ancient Greece and contemporary America. London: Duckworth; 2009.
11. Schechner R. Rasaesthetics. The Drama Review. 2001;45:27–50.
12. Moreno JL. Psychodrama, vol. 3. Beacon, NY: Beacon House; 1969.
13. Bielańska A. Monodrama as a specific intervention in the treatment of auditory hallucinations. Psychoterapia. 2016;1:29–42.
14. Meisner S, Longwell D. Sanford Meisner on acting. New York, NY: Random House; 1987.
15. Panero ME. A psychological exploration of the experience of acting. Creativity Research Journal. 2019;31:428–42.
16. Boal A. Theatre of the oppressed. New York, NY: Theatre Communications Group; 1979.
17. Johnson DR, Emunah R. Current approaches in drama therapy. Springfield, IL: Charles C. Thomas; 2009.
18. Austin SF. Principles of drama-therapy: a handbook for dramatists. New York, NY: Sopherim; 1917.
19. Jones P. An analysis of the first articulation of drama therapy: Austin's 'Principles of drama-therapy: a handbook for dramatists' (1917). The Arts in Psychotherapy. 2013;40:352–7.
20. Slade P. Child drama. London: University Press; 1954.

21. Jennings S. Remedial drama. London: Pitman; 1974.
22. Jennings S. Dramatherapy: theory and practice for teachers and clinicians. London: Routledge; 1987.
23. Jennings S. Dramatherapy with families, groups and individuals: waiting in the wings. London: Jessica Kingsley; 1990.
24. Jennings S. Introduction to dramatherapy: Ariadne's ball of thread. London: Jessica Kingsley; 1997.
25. Jennings S. Healthy attachments and neuro-dramatic-play. London: Jessica Kingsley; 2010.
26. Hougham R, Jones B. Dramatherapy: reflections and praxis. London: Palgrave Macmillan; 2017.
27. Gersie A. Storymaking in education and therapy. London: Jessica Kingsley; 1990.
28. Schattner G, Courtney R. Drama in therapy. New York, NY: Drama Book Specialists; 1981.
29. Emunah R. Acting for real: drama therapy process, technique, and performance. New York, NY: Routledge; 2019.
30. Landy R. Persona and performance--the meaning of role in drama, therapy and everyday life. New York, NY: Guilford; 1993.
31. Landy R. Role theory and the role method of drama therapy. In: Johnson D, Emunah R, editors. Current approaches in drama therapy. Springfield, IL: Charles C. Thomas; 2009.
32. World Alliance of Drama Therapy. Associations and representatives. 2019. www.worldallianceofdramatherapy.com. Accessed 2 Dec 2019.
33. Pendzik S. On dramatic reality and its therapeutic function in drama therapy. The Arts in Psychotherapy. 2006;33:271–80.
34. Cassidy S, Gumley A, Turnbull S. Safety, play, enablement, and active involvement: themes from a grounded theory study of practitioner and client experiences of change processes in dramatherapy. The Arts in Psychotherapy. 2017;55:174–85.
35. Cox M. Shakespeare comes to Broadmoor. London: Jessica Kingsley; 1992.
36. Emunah R. Drama therapy with adult psychiatric patients. The Arts in Psychotherapy. 1983;10:77–84.
37. Langley D, Langley G. Drama therapy and psychiatry. New York, NY: Routledge; 2018.
38. Sajnani N. The implicated witness: towards a relational aesthetic in dramatherapy. Dramatherapy. 2012;34:6–21.
39. Sajnani N, Johnson DR. Trauma-informed drama therapy: transforming clinics, classrooms, and communities. Springfield, IL: Charles C. Thomas; 2014.
40. Forrester AM, Johnson DR. The role of dramatherapy in an extremely short-term in-patient psychiatric unit. In: Gersie A, editor. Brief treatment approaches to drama therapy. London: Routledge; 1995. p. 125–38.
41. Reynolds A. Developmental transformations: improvisational drama therapy with children in acute inpatient psychiatry. Social Work with Groups. 2011;34:296–309.
42. Ron Y. Psychodrama's role in alleviating acute distress: a case study of an open therapy group in an inpatient psychiatry ward. Frontiers in Psychology. 2018;9:2075. https://www.ncbi.nlm.nih.gov/pmc/articles/PMC6218611/.
43. Butler J. Playing with madness: developmental transformations and the treatment of schizophrenia. The Arts in Psychotherapy. 2012;39:87–94.
44. Emunah R, Johnson DR. The impact of theatrical performance on the self-images of psychiatric patients. The Arts in Psychotherapy. 1983;10:233–9.
45. Sajnani N, Cho A, Landis H, Raucher G, Trytan N. Collaborative discourse analysis on the use of drama therapy to treat depression in adults. In: Zubala A, Karkou V, editors. Arts therapies in the treatment of depression. New York, NY: Routledge; 2018. p. 87–101.
46. McMullian S, Burch D. 'I am more than my disease': an embodied approach to understanding clinical populations using Landy's Taxonomy of roles in concert with the DSM-5. Drama Therapy Review. 2017;3:29–43.
47. McAdam E, Johnson DR. Reducing depressive symptoms in adolescents with posttraumatic stress disorder using drama therapy. In: Zubala A, Karkou V, editors. Arts therapies in the treatment of depression. New York, NY: Routledge; 2018. p. 48–67.

48. Pitre R, Sajnani N, Johnson DR. Trauma-centered developmental transformations as exposure treatment for young children. Drama Therapy Review. 2015;1:41–54.
49. Ruddy R, Dent-Brown K. Drama therapy for schizophrenia or schizophrenia-like illnesses. Cochrane Database of Systematic Reviews. 2007;(1):CD005378. https://doi.org/10.1002/14651858.CD005378.pub2.
50. Casson J. Drama, psychotherapy and psychosis: dramatherapy and psychodrama with people who hear voices. New York, NY: Brunner-Routledge; 2004.
51. Johnson DR. Drama therapy and the schizophrenic condition. In: Schattner G, Courtney R, editors. Drama in therapy. New York, NY: Drama Book Specialists; 1981. p. 47–64.
52. Johnson DR. The representation of the internal world in catatonic schizophrenia. Psychiatry. 1984;47:299–314.
53. Crawford MJ, Patterson S. Arts therapies for people with schizophrenia: an emerging evidence base. Evidence Based Mental Health. 2007;10:69–70.
54. Sancar F, Şahin S, Şahin G, Eren N. The assessment of a drama therapy process for patients with severe psychiatric patients. European Psychiatry. 2017;41:S615.
55. Anari A, Ddadsetan, Sedghpour BS. The effectiveness of drama therapy on decreasing the symptoms of social anxiety disorder in children. European Psychiatry. 2019;24:514.
56. Klees S. A hero's journey in a German psychiatric hospital: a case study on the use of role method in individual drama therapy. Drama Therapy Review. 2016;2:99–110.
57. Moran GS, Alon U. Playback theatre and recovery in mental health: preliminary evidence. The Arts in Psychotherapy. 2011;38:318–24.
58. Dunphy K, Baker F, Dumaresq E, Carroll-Haskins K, Eikholt J, Ercole M, Kaimal G, Meyer K, Sajnani N, Shamir O, Wosch T. Creative arts interventions to address depression in older adults: a systematic review of outcomes, processes and mechanisms. Frontiers in Psychology. 2019;9:2655. https://doi.org/10.3389/fpsyg.2018.02655.
59. Keulen-de Vos M, van den Broek E, Bernstein DP, Vallentin R, Arntz A. Evoking emotional states in personality disordered offenders: an experimental pilot study of experiential drama therapy techniques. The Arts in Psychotherapy. 2017;53:80–8.
60. Smeijsters H, Cleven G. The treatment of aggression using arts therapies in forensic psychiatry: results of a qualitative inquiry. The Arts in Psychotherapy. 2006;33:37–58.
61. Orkibi H, Bar N, Eliakim I. The effect of drama-based group therapy on aspects of mental illness stigma. The Arts in Psychotherapy. 2014;41:458–66.
62. Yotis L, Theocharopoulos C, Fragiadaki C, Begioglou D. Using playback theatre to address the stigma of mental disorders. The Arts in Psychotherapy. 2017;55:80–4.

18 Drama/Theatre Practice in Psychiatric Care

Paul N. Animbom

The practice of drama and theatre in the context of psychiatric care is age-old. It spans from ancient ritual performances in African traditions to Aristotle's emphasis on the cathartic effect of tragedy. Drama and theatre techniques have been employed throughout human history to improve people's well-being with different appellations such as dramatherapy (drama therapy in American English). While many studies on the importance of dramatherapy to human development have been carried out, few are committed to examining the impact on psychiatric care. Nisha Sajnani's study on dramatherapy in this context is relevant for providing the historical perspective and therapeutic mechanisms used as well as treatment guidelines. It complements a study carried out by Paul Animbom on therapeutic theatre: an experience from a mental clinic in Yaoundé Cameroon [1] which brought out the impact of drama and theatre techniques with inpatient and outpatient psychiatric participants.

The chapter presents a history of the use of dramatic processes to promote well-being among peoples from Africa, Asia, and later on, Europe that were principally drawn from healing rituals. This section exposes some of the key practitioners that were involved in implementing drama-based techniques in health. This practice dates as far back as 500–300 BC with Bharatmuni's Natyashastra and in 335 BC with Aristotle's *Poetics* as concerns theories; Jung, Reich, Moreno, Growtowski, Stanislavski, and Boal as concern practitioners of the contemporary period. Worth noting also is the introduction of the use of drama-based techniques in psychiatric care by Vladimir Iljine as early as 1908–1917 when he applied it to his patients and

P. N. Animbom (✉)
Centre for Research and Practice of Art Related Therapy,
Yaoundé, Cameroon

Department of Performing and Visual Arts, The University of Bamenda,
Bamenda, Cameroon

Department of Arts and Cultural Studies, University of Copenhagen,
Copenhagen, Denmark

U. Volpe (ed.), *Arts Therapies in Psychiatric Rehabilitation*,
https://doi.org/10.1007/978-3-030-76208-7_18

emphasis was laid on spontaneity, flexibility, expressivity, sensitivity, and the ability to communicate [2]. The key in all these is that, there is a systematic recognition of the importance of using drama and theatre activities in the upkeep of psychiatric patients.

The emergence of the field of dramatherapy (which is a relatively new approach of drama and theatre-based methods in psychiatry) marks a turning point in psychiatric care. Sajnani again shows that dramatherapy is interdisciplinary; combining theatrical and psychological orientations. Practiced in more than 30 countries worldwide, dramatherapy provides people with a safe and secure experience that facilitates emotional stability and creative expression through playful, dramatic activities. Positive cognitive and behavioral changes, self-awareness, perspective-taking, improved interpersonal skills, enhanced emotional expression, and modulation are key therapeutic benefits of dramatherapy in psychiatric care.

For dramatherapy to achieve therapeutic outcomes in psychiatric care, some basic principles must be respected. In this light, Sajnani draws a connecting line between the four main areas that preoccupy dramatherapists: brief acute inpatient care, long-term inpatient care, outpatient care, and staff development. Though the African sector is still lagging behind on the full implementation of dramatherapy in psychiatric care (most particularly in hospitals), South Africa and Cameroon are implementing some relative aspects of drama and theatre-based techniques for mental and emotional development in community settings [3, 4]. No matter where it is practiced, dramatherapy basically involves warm up, focusing, main activity, closure and de-rolling, and completion. This notwithstanding, Sajnani highlights an important facet of dramatherapy in this chapter which many scholars/practitioners fail to develop. This is the inclusion of dramatic projection within the traditional talk psychotherapy. In this process, inner feelings, fears, and wishes are concretized within a fictionalized role or inanimate objects such as a figurine, mask, puppet, or text are used to externalize unconscious processes and clarify hidden truths about self.

It goes without doubt that dramatherapy is effective in psychiatric care in Western and African settings. As evidenced in the abovementioned study carried out in a mental health clinic in Yaoundé-Cameroon, it was noted that acting and engaging in therapeutic theatre activities provides an intense pleasure which permits the discovery of parts of oneself which hitherto were unknown. It enables the participants to explore different states of being as well as the nuances of their sentiments. They make use of their bodies, voices, and all other human potentials. In this way, drama and theatre bring into play physical and psychological mechanisms that promote mental and emotional well-being in a group setting or individual setup. According to Landy [5] when the relationship process in the group works, the participant-actors discover ways to engage more deeply with the theme. Their relationship deepens, shifts, and changes.

Through active participation in the therapeutic process, the participants in psychiatric care achieve self-liberation. Their inhibitions and self-doubts gradually disappear as they dialogue with other participants. Through this, self-identification, self-esteem, self-recognition as people capable of changing their destinies, and self-reliance are embedded in their sub-consciences.

The use of dramatherapy in mental health in partnership with other approaches in the context of psychiatric care blends well with the notion of co-creation. The aim of dramatherapy hereby becomes an opportunity to build the participants' personal and developmental skills and produce therapeutic effects and affects. Though still ignored by many in Cameroon and Africa under the westernized appellation, this therapeutic paradigm can be seen as an attempt to fill the gap that exists in the domain of mental health when it comes to psychiatric care. The African setting is one with particular sociocultural and diverse environmental settings that requires particular measures and methods to be used. In this regard, a community-based approach to dramatherapy can be used since health in this postcolonial setting is still considered a community, not an individual affair. In the practice, participants' opinions and perspectives on the problems handled in each workshop are taken into consideration in a process involving collective creation geared towards the quest for change. Community-based dramatherapy within psychiatric care offers a special means to unite, uplift, teach, inspire, heal, and foster change and well-being. It is a contextualized creative art therapy applicable in psychiatric care in which participants attend a deeper understanding of their psychological states and develop coping mechanisms and readaptation skills vis-à-vis mental health.

References

1. Animbom NP. Therapeutic theatre: an experience from a mental health clinic in Yaoundé-Cameroon. Arts Health. 2017;9(3):269–78.
2. Jones P. Drama as therapy. Theatre as living. London: Routledge; 1996.
3. Animbom NP. Culture and mental health: an evaluation of *Esie* performance as a community-based approach of dramatherapy in Cameroon. In: Jennings S, Holmwood C, editors. Routledge International handbook of Dramatherapy. London: Routledge; 2016. p. 36–45.
4. Animbom NP, editor. Participatory theatre and therapy. Beau Bassin: EUE; 2019.
5. Landy R. Waiting for therapeutic theatre: a search for a new form of drama therapy, Couch and Stage. 2013. http://www.psychologytoday.com/blog/couch-and-stage/201305/waiting-therapeutic-theatre. Accessed 28 Jun 2013.

19 Drama Therapy and Psychiatric Care in India: Practice and Potential

Maitri Gopalakrishna

Dr. Sajnani's chapter offers a sound introduction to drama therapy in the context of psychiatric care. In this commentary, I specifically look at the potential and practice of drama therapy in the Indian context with case examples to illustrate the versatility and adaptability of this therapeutic methodology.

India suffers from a large care-gap in mental health. Published estimates of numbers of psychiatrists in the entire country range from 4000 to 9000. This is well below desirable for a population of 1.3 billion. In addition, there is a gross imbalance of distribution of these practitioners across the country with a few urban centres commanding most resources [1–3]. The stigma against seeking psychiatric care in India is also documented [4, 5].

In a context such as this, the role of non-psychiatrist mental health practitioners is very significant. Psychiatric social workers, clinical psychologists and psychotherapists have now become a more ubiquitous part of treatment teams in India. While non-governmental organisations in India have recognised the value of drama therapy in community-based mental health and rehabilitation work for some time now [6], psychiatric/neuroscience facilities have taken their time. Only recently, a few psychiatric/neuroscience facilities in the country, such as Fortis and VIMHANS hospitals in Delhi, have included arts therapists as part of their teams. Individual psychiatrists are also beginning to refer patients specifically for arts therapies to support psychopharmacological treatment.

There is a growing recognition of the potential of the arts therapies and specifically drama therapy both within and outside clinical contexts in India. A therapy that includes non-verbal processes can be effective in the Indian cultural context where "talking" about one's emotions is quite alien. Drama therapy is well suited to groups, which can make it useful for larger community settings and in situations where an issue may be socially situated as well. The stigma against accessing traditional mental health services in India can be sidestepped by placing the therapeutic

M. Gopalakrishna (✉)
Parivarthan Counselling Training and Research Centre, Bengaluru, Karnataka, India

U. Volpe (ed.), *Arts Therapies in Psychiatric Rehabilitation*,
https://doi.org/10.1007/978-3-030-76208-7_19

work in an artistic/creative container. Finally, drama therapy makes the space for the integration of specific cultural material into the work such as stories, mythology, songs, or symbols [7].

However, the number of professionally trained arts therapists in India is low and includes few drama therapists. In 2019, the small community of drama therapists in India came together for the first time to run an experiential symposium for other mental health practitioners at the National Institute of Mental Health and Neurosciences in Bangalore. Soon after, we created the Drama Therapy India collective. We are now beginning to explore training programmes, professional associations and research in order to grow, regulate and streamline the field.

I have practiced as a drama therapist in India for the last 12 years. In my clinical individual work, I embed drama therapy methods within traditional talk therapy. The guiding theoretical threads and approaches that inform my practice include intersectional feminist therapy (recognising the role of systemic oppressions in psychological suffering), role theory (that proposes that human personality and behaviour can be understood as arising from a dynamic tension between a cluster of socially performed roles), narrative approaches (the power of narrativizations and the possibility of re-authoring) and dialectical behaviour therapy (a system of psychosocial skills building).

Here is a case example to illustrate what this could look like. One of my clients was a man in his early 30s who was receiving psychopharmacological treatment for generalized anxiety disorder and had been through one inpatient hospitalization. He began working with me soon after his discharge. His psychiatrist continued to monitor his mediation. My work with him involved several iterative processes. We worked on recognising signs of overwhelm as sensations in his body and responding to those using specific movements, in order for him to build and practice embodied emotion regulation skills. He worked on his relationship with his anxiety by using aesthetic tools to create distance and re-author his associations with it. Then, he worked on his own identity as being more than just the anxious one. He was able to conceptualize the different aspects of himself and exercise choice in what role he played in a given context. We also worked through images and metaphors to be able to process traumatic events of the past in a safe way. The work continued for a year. While the anxiety did not disappear completely, it seemed to be less present, less significant and more manageable for him. It has been 3 years since our first session. He has not had another hospital admission to date.

It is important for psychological therapy to be cognisant of sociopolitical structures of inequality and oppression as well as cultural specificities of the contexts we work in. Many of my colleagues in the arts therapies in India do this consciously through participatory curriculum development for training and advocacy, incorporating indigenous art forms and practices into community-based or clinical work and so on [8–12]. For instance, when using drama therapy processes and therapeutic theatre with a group of women who were working through the trauma of having been sexually abused as children, processes of personal suffering and social complicity had to be explored in tandem. Dramatic forms were used to link, juxtapose and work through these processes simultaneously [13]. Participants reported the following as the most transformative factors of the process: (1) the collaborative group aspect, (2) being able to interrogate problematic social beliefs and having access to alternate discourses, (3) privileging the body by working in action and (4) doing serious work with creativity, aestheticism and even humour [7].

As is evident from the chapter by Dr. Sajnani, drama therapy today has Eurocentric roots. As a way of expanding the foundations of the field, Dr. Sajnani and I are researching the *Natya*sastra, an ancient Indian treatise on performance. Part of our research is theoretical. The rest is practice-based to see how conventions and methods within the *Natyashastra* could contribute to our work as drama therapists and trainers. I have experimented with teaching clients specific breath and body patterns (drawn from *Natyashastra*-based performance technique) for emotion regulation. While clients have reported these methods as being helpful, further research is needed to test the efficacy of these techniques [14].

There is great potential for drama therapy in the treatment of psychiatric concerns in India, provided care is taken to understand its specific sociopolitical and cultural context.

References

1. Garg K, Kumar CN, Chandra PS. Number of psychiatrists in India: baby steps forward, but a long way to go. Indian J Psychiatry. 2019;61(1):104–5.
2. Gururaj G, Varghese M, Benegal V, Rao GN, Pathak K, Singh LK, et al. National Mental Health Survey of India, 2015–16: prevalence, patterns and outcomes. Bangalore: National Institute of Mental Health and Neuro Sciences Publication No. 129; 2016. p. 90–121.
3. Kaur R, Pathak RK. Treatment gap in mental healthcare: reflections from policy and research. Econ Polit Week. 2017;L11(31):34–40.
4. Gaiha SM, Sunil GA, Kumar R, Menon S. Enhancing mental health literacy in India to reduce stigma: the fountainhead to improve help-seeking behaviour. J Public Ment Health. 2014;13(3).
5. Srivastava K, Chatterjee K, Bhat PS. Mental health awareness: the Indian scenario. Ind Psychiatry J. 2016;25(2):131–4.
6. Casson J. Dramatherapy in India. Dramatherapy. 1993;15(3):17–21.
7. Gopalakrishna M. Pliable and playable: drama therapy, women's narratives and childhood sexual abuse. Unpublished PhD thesis. Tata Institute of Social Sciences, Mumbai, India; 2018.
8. Chabukswar A, Balsara Z. Converging lineages arts-based therapy in contemporary India. In: Jennings S, Holmwood C, editors. The Routledge international handbook of Dramatherapy. London: Routledge; 2016. p. 19–25.
9. Chakrabarti O. Genesis of a new cultural model: envisioning the scope for art therapy in India—a pioneering journey. In: Hougham R, Pitruzzella S, Scoble S, editors. Cultural landscapes in the arts therapies. London: ECArTE Publication, University of Plymouth Press; 2018. p. 217–35.
10. Jhaveri K. Healing roots of indigenous crafts: adapting traditions of India for art therapy practice. In: Leone L, editor. Craft in art therapy: diverse approaches to the transformative power of craft materials and methods. London: Routledge; 2020. Forthcoming.
11. Kashyap T. My body my wisdom: a handbook of creative dance therapy. New Delhi: Penguin Books; 2005.
12. Zhou TY, Kim N, Machida S, Sakiyama Y, Tsai P, Lee T, Ho RTH, Bijlani R, Mehta D, Bui M. Dance movement therapy in Asia: an overview of the profession and its practice. Creat Arts Educ Ther. 2019;5(1):40–50.

13. Gopalakrishna M, Rao S. Performance, revelation and resistance: interweaving the artistic and the therapeutic in devised theatre. Indian Theatre J. 2017;1(1):83–90.
14. Sajnani N, Gopalakrishna M. Rasa: exploring the influence of Indian performance theory in drama therapy. Drama Ther Rev. 2017;3(2):225–40.

Facilitating Empathy Through Drama Therapy for Clients and Clinicians Across the Spectrum of Psychiatric Care

20

Dana George Trottier

In her chapter, Dr. Sajnani provides an expansive journey through the available literature and research on drama therapy in the context of psychiatric care. Sajnani invites the reader to consider the historical narrative of drama therapy as a field as well as basic principles and techniques, before organizing the findings across four distinct areas of psychiatric care: brief acute inpatient, long-term inpatient, outpatient, and staff development. Sajnani concludes with a call to action to expand the body of knowledge in these areas to research practices and increase access to creative approaches.

Before placing Sajnani's chapter into a broader context of my own experience and research, I want to share the lens through which I reviewed this chapter. For 10 years, I have had the privilege to work as a drama therapist in a public hospital system in New York City with an established and expanding creative arts therapy program that currently employs over 120 creative arts therapists across the spectrum of psychiatric care. Additionally, I have utilized my approach as a drama therapist to design curriculum for staff development, training, and clinical supervision. Moreover, I teach a course at New York University entitled Drama Therapy for Clinical Populations. As a result, I am deeply interested and invested in the role that drama therapy plays in the treatment of individuals and groups in psychiatric care.

Out of the number of outcomes from drama therapy Sajnani mentions, the one of most interest to me and my work today is that of empathy. In my experience, facilitating empathy through drama therapy is at the core of psychiatric rehabilitation and a necessary component across the spectrum of care. As Sajnani indicates in this chapter, drama therapy can be utilized to "temporarily suspend the plausible in order to explore the possible." If we apply this same notion to the way a drama

D. G. Trottier (✉)
Behavioral Health Services, NYC Health + Hospitals/Kings County and Simulation Center, Brookyln, NY, USA

Program in Drama Therapy, New York University, New York, NY, USA
e-mail: dgt219@nyu.edu

U. Volpe (ed.), *Arts Therapies in Psychiatric Rehabilitation*,
https://doi.org/10.1007/978-3-030-76208-7_20

therapist takes in the treatment space and the individuals who perform within them, then we can begin to understand how a drama therapist facilitates empathy. When encountering clients in psychiatric care, I utilize my lens as a drama therapist to understand the way in which the client and their behavior performs in the treatment space—the metaphorical stage [1]. For example, a client who presents with active psychosis and verbally responds to internal stimuli may engage the clinician in a soliloquy, monologue, or dialogue, depending on their current experience with symptoms. Assessing their current performance helps me to understand my role in relationship and illuminates a dialogical point of entry into treatment planning.

By contextualizing the behavior of the client as performance, I am able to shift my notion of *as-is* to *as-if*. A first step in understanding a client is accepting their current performance *as if* it is an adaptable behavior that has been developed or acquired over time to support the client's efforts in living the best they can in the social world, or the *as is*. Given the relational potential of empathy, by stepping into the world of the client first, I can facilitate the cocreation of consensus reality. A drama therapist journeys alongside the client to come to an understanding of the origin and function of the symptoms and behaviors and to discover alternate ways to live with and live beyond their identified symptoms.

For example, I recently worked with a young adult, who I will refer to as Sarah, who spoke of our group treatment as "classes" and her peers on the unit as her "classmates"; what is more, she assigned each peer a prescriptive character style that matched stereotypical roles in high school: the jock, the popular girl, the nerd. Sarah's efforts in contextualizing her experience in the frame of school was her attempt at organizing and digesting her own understanding of being in the hospital, as well as repairing her own experiences with bullying. Her ability to adjust to her environment in this way was a testament to her creativity, adaptability, and insight, not a psychotic process. When Sarah transitioned from inpatient care to an outpatient program, the clinicians initially noted that Sarah demonstrated regressive behaviors that may be indicative of readmission. Upon further investigation, I discovered that the clinicians were attempting to reorganize Sarah's understanding of the outpatient program as group treatment, rather than the metaphor of school. The clinicians were attempting to shift Sarah's worldview too far beyond her own readiness, into a realm that was no longer cocreated, and instead based on the clinics desire for performed insight. When I consulted with the team on the change in behavior, I shared with them the necessity of viewing the environment through Sarah's eyes to step into her world—a safe space she established for herself where healing was possible. As their perspectives joined, and empathy entered the relationship, Sarah was able to successfully complete the program and "graduate" to an even lower level of care.

As a clinical supervisor and educator, my research has focused on the use of embodied supervision to enhance empathy and understanding. By taking a moment to step into the shoes of their client through embodiment and performance, the therapist is able to connect the outer performance of the client to their inner world [2]. At present, I utilize simulation methodologies and embodiment to teach interdisciplinary teams how to respond to crisis situations that may arise on the unit, or in the clinic. Through intentional role-playing of crisis situations in a training environment, clinicians are able to play out the role of the client to build embodied empathy, and to try out interventions as clinicians to build muscle memory for when crisis may perform in the treatment space [3]. Embodied supervision supports the development of embodied empathy and therapist role responsiveness to expand the capacity of the therapist to respond to the varying needs of the individuals across the spectrum of psychiatric care.

I have suggested that utilizing drama therapy to facilitate empathy is a crucial aspect of treatment in psychiatric rehabilitation. Shifting from narrative retelling to a here and now performance, drama therapy shifts the learning by integrating the mind and body, where life and practice can be rehearsed *as if* the moment is taking place in the present. As psychiatric rehabilitation continues to expand beyond the medical model towards a person-centered model, drama therapy contributes pathways to empathy to support both clients and clinicians in cocreating, collaborative approaches to care.

References

1. Trottier DG. Therapist as guide: role profiles, metaphor, and story to understand the parallel journey of the queer therapist and the straight client. In: MacWilliam B, Harris BT, Trottier DG, Long K, editors. Creative arts therapies and the LGBTQ community: theory and practice. London: Jessica Kingsley; 2019a. p. 75–100.
2. Trottier DG, Hilt L. I don't feel naked: the use of embodied supervision to examine the impact of patient clothing on clinical countertransference on an inpatient psychiatry unit. Drama Ther Rev. 2017;3:261–83.
3. Trottier D. Embodied empathy: utilizing drama therapy techniques in crisis management [conference session]. In: Creative arts therapies conference: transforming care & wellness across our health system. New York: NYC Health + Hospitals/Gouverneur; 2019b.

Empirical Research Considerations in Drama Therapy: A Response Essay

21

Laura L. Wood

As Sajnani mentions at the close of her essay, the profession of drama therapy must provide empirical research for professional advancement. Not only would empirical research allow drama therapy to continue growing as a credible form of mental health intervention and treatment internationally, but in some geographical contexts (such as the United States of America) empirical evidence is required in securing third-party payor reimbursement [1]. This brief essay will review drama therapy research in an empirical context, discuss the value of considering manualization, and suggest specific research tracks that could help elevate the profession.

Armstrong et al. [2] provided a comprehensive literature review of empirical drama therapy research. They defined empirical research as "the derivation of knowledge about drama therapy and related processes/techniques from direct or indirect observation or experience" (p. 3), and the authors included arts-based, qualitative, and quantitative methodologies. The authors reviewed 89 articles and found the current state of drama therapy research could be categorized into three broad themes: studies about drama therapy interventions/assessments, drama therapy studies as applied to special populations, and the profession of drama therapy. The authors highlighted that while the articles do show enthusiasm, promise, and help make visible the profession, there is also not one approach in drama therapy that has a significant body of research knowledge.

Armstrong et al. [3] built on the aforementioned literature review with an article that analyzed 44 of the drama therapy articles that aimed to provide direct information regarding the effectiveness of drama therapy intervention. The authors found 14 themes that the empirical studies could be categorized in: emotional and behavioral symptoms, self-confidence and self-esteem, self-expression, well-being, emotional regulation, empathy, academic performance, language and linguistic performance,

L. L. Wood (✉)
Division of Expressive Therapies, Lesley University, Cambridge, MA, USA
e-mail: lwood5@lesley.edu

U. Volpe (ed.), *Arts Therapies in Psychiatric Rehabilitation*,
https://doi.org/10.1007/978-3-030-76208-7_21

stigma, bodily awareness, empowerment, and spontaneity. While these domains are quite promising for the profession of drama therapy, and certainly have meaningful applications in regard to psychiatric rehabilitation, the authors also articulated some limitations. One issue was sample size. The authors indicated that 70% of the studies had 20 or less participants and many were contextualized as pilot studies. Another major concern the authors had was that preliminary research in drama therapy tended to not scaffold into more expansive work, but rather work as small standalone studies, which leaves the profession without a meaningful way of "building on our own body of pre-existing research" (p. 179).

One potential solution towards an empirical evidence base would be to manualize aspects of drama therapy and to study the outcomes. While manualization does not necessarily equate to a better form of treatment, it does ensure a protocol that can be studied and replicated to allow for a meaningful base of research to be developed [4].

The CoActive Therapeutic Theater (CoATT) model is the first manualized model of therapeutic theater, a form of drama therapy. The CoATT model is a 14-week process designed to work with persons in various forms of recovery such as eating disorders, substance use disorders, or medical recovery [5]. The creators of the model, two registered drama therapists in North America, envisioned the process as a stepping stone between higher levels of care and more independent levels of care. The model consists of seven "movements." Each movement has an identified goal that is linked to specific drama therapy exercises culminating in a public performance that explores recovery. Participants are asked to answer the question: "What is a theme of recovery you would like to explore through performance to strengthen your own recovery and to share with an audience?" The work is metaphorical, rather than autobiographical, and reported outcomes have included increased spontaneity, mental flexibility, and self-confidence, reduction of eating disorder/substance use behaviors, and experiencing self as an agent of change in the community [5–7].

While all forms of research are valuable and necessary, working towards measurable processes and outcomes will likely be needed for the future of drama therapy to grow in numbers and be accepted as a mainstream form of clinical mental health treatment. Future research might consider building on pilot study data currently available, pairing aforementioned outcomes noted in Armstrong et al. [2, 3] with already developed reliable and valid measures, or progressing one's clinical drama therapy practice towards manualization. Additionally, as major research continues to emerge in neuroscience, trauma, and the body [8–10], drama therapists pairing their work and concepts alongside these disciplines could provide valuable interdisciplinary collaboration and exciting new outcomes. Finally, ensuring that manualized treatments consider addresssing systemic issues and are developed with cultural sensitivity is essential in continuing to dismantle structual oppression [11].

References

1. Hatchett GT. Monitoring the counseling relationship and client progress as alternatives to prescriptive empirically supported therapies. J Ment Health Couns. 2017;39(2):104–15.
2. Armstrong CR, Frydman JS, Rowe C. A snapshot of empirical drama therapy research: conducting a general review of the literature. M.Sm. der empirischen Dramatherapieforschung. 2019a.
3. Armstrong CR, Frydman JS, Wood S. Prominent themes in drama therapy effectiveness research. Drama Ther Rev. 2019b;5(2):173–216.
4. Truijens F, Zühlke-van Hulzen L, Vanheule S. To manualize, or not to manualize: is that still the question? A systematic review of empirical evidence for manual superiority in psychological treatment. J Clin Psychol. 2019;75(3):329–43.
5. Wood LL, Mowers D. The co-active therapeutic theatre model: a manualized approach to creating therapeutic theatre with persons in recovery. Drama Ther Rev. 2019;5(2):217–34.
6. Wood LL, Bryant D, Scirocco K, Datta H, Alimonti S, Mowers D. Aphasia Park: a pilot study using the co-active therapeutic theater model with clients in aphasia recovery. Arts Psychother. 2020;67:101611.
7. Wood LL. The use of therapeutic theater in supporting clients in eating disorder recovery after intensive treatment: a qualitative study; 2016.
8. Ogden P, Minton K, Pain C. Trauma and the body: a sensorimotor approach to psychotherapy (Norton series on interpersonal neurobiology). New York: WW Norton; 2006.
9. Siegel DJ. Pocket guide to interpersonal neurobiology: an integrative handbook of the mind (Norton series on interpersonal neurobiology). New York: WW Norton; 2012.
10. Van der Kolk BA. The body keeps the score: brain, mind, and body in the healing of trauma. New York: Penguin Books; 2015.
11. Sajnani N. The critical turn towards evidence in drama therapy. Drama Ther Rev. 2019;5(2):169–72.

22 Healing Aspects of Drama and Theatre and Perspectives in Dramatherapy

Elisabetta Denti

The intentional use of healing aspects of drama and theatre as a therapeutic process is globally known as dramatherapy (BADT). In Italy, we have not yet managed to build a common identity for the therapeutic approach to theatrical mediation, and therefore two disciplines known under the terms of "theatretherapy" and "dramatherapy" coexist substantially. They have both been recognized through the approval of law no. 4/2013 (provisions relating to professions not organized in orders and colleges) which governs art therapy.

The Italian Federation of Theatretherapy (FIT) defines itself as "an association of professionals who target different social spheres (...) who take care and support people with mental and physical discomfort, using theater workshops with body mediation and spontaneity in order to educate to perception, improve the relationship with oneself, bringing out one's human potential."

The Italian Professional Society of Dramatherapy (SPID) defines drama therapy as "artistic therapy based on dramatic arts and applied to clinical, educational and social, training and personal development contexts, both individually and as a group" [1].

There are differences in terms of the theoretical reference system and consequently in the context of the application paradigms, since each discipline has a different historical and cultural panorama. However, they are united by the substantial use of the same instruments (body, voice, stage and transitional space, game, and mediating objects of theatrical art) and are oriented towards common objectives [2].

Dramatherapy considers the body as an excellent therapeutic tool. The process is born, grows, and develops through the body. The therapist's body is defined by Roussillon as a "malleable medium" [3]. Its main characteristics, proposed for the first time by Milner and subsequently developed by Roussillon, are indestructibility,

E. Denti (✉)
Riabilitatori Associati, Milan, Italy

U. Volpe (ed.), *Arts Therapies in Psychiatric Rehabilitation*,
https://doi.org/10.1007/978-3-030-76208-7_22

extreme sensitivity, the possibility of transformation, unconditional availability, and its own animation. It is through the body and its characteristics that all perceptions are realized and become possible. In his major work, Merleau-Ponty considers sensitivity as an activity that structures sensory stimuli, configures them, and invests them with meaning [4]. This perceptual process occurs in vivo in a dramatherapeutic setting. The reflection on the body is intertwined with the use of the voice in dramatherapy. Attigui considers the voice as the instrument that allows to explore the concrete nature of the transitional space [5]. The theatrical space, inhabited by the body and animated by the voice, thus becomes the place of representation.

Rehabilitation conceives space (and time) not only as a real and objective parameter but considers it as a place (and moment) of personal and subjective possibility, a space of distance and proximity that allows perspectives, movement, and representation. The scenic space is the place of the therapeutic relationship that takes place over time. In order to fully introduce the reflection on dramatherapy, it is essential to introduce the peculiar concept that is proper to this mediation that is illusory stage space. This is part of the clinical application of the theater between the subject's imaginary internal space and the external real space. To build this space, it is essential to enter a unique space, special for rules, for the emotional state that underlies and supports it, in order to build a relational path that allows you to put in place exercises useful to build a state of play. The space of existential choice is in fact the space of the limit. This transitional space represents the possibility of escaping the space of existential choice, where each act implies real consequences and judgment, and entering the dimension of the possibility in which the subject, and in particular the carriers of psychic discomfort, can be free to express parts of alternative, unknown selves by playing. So, they do not incur in the consequences that the real expressive act could imply on a concrete or intrapsychic level. The play corresponds to the driving force of experience. Mediation objects such as, by way of non-exhaustive example, puppets, the use of theatrical text or creative writing techniques, represent possibilities and tools that a dramatherapist can use to animate the playful experience. The analysis of the function of inanimate objects in the process of self-representation of the psyche and self-awareness is a perspective that Roussillon proposes to fully understand the process just described [6].

In conclusion, it is clear that in order to have the adequate tools for dramatherapy it is important to know the potential of this mediation that can be acquired through a serious and constant training path. In order to be able to use them in a coherent and functional way, it is essential to know the characteristics of the people we are addressing to and to establish work objectives shared by the client and by the group of work colleagues [1]. Working with competence and professionalism can reveal wonderful and unexpected perspectives.

References

1. Volpe U, Facchini D, Magnotti R, Diamare S, Denti E, Viganò CA. Le arti-terapie nel contesto della riabilitazione psicosociale in Italia. Psichiatria e Psicoterapia. 2016;35(4):170–4.

2. Vita A, Dell'Osso L, Mucci A. Manuale di clinica e riabilitazione psichiatrica. Dalle conoscenze teoriche alla pratica dei servizi di salute mentale, vol. 2. Rome: Giovanni Fioriti; 2019. p. 739.
3. Roussillon R. Le jeu et l'entre-jeu. Paris: Le fil rouge; 2012.
4. Merleau-Ponty M. Phénoménologie de la perception. Paris: Gallimard; 1945.
5. Attigui P. De l'illusion théatrale à l'espace thérapeutique. Jeu, transfert, psychose. Paris: Dunod; 2012.
6. Roussillon R. L'objet « médium malléable » et la conscience de soi. Dans l'Autre. 2001;2:241–54.

23 Challenges of Research in Drama Therapy

Simone Klees

Nisha Sajnani gives an insight into basic principles of drama therapy and shows that in the young research field of drama therapy there are studies that describe the effects of drama therapy interventions in different areas of psychiatric care. The chapter shows that for reasons outlined by Sajnani, drama therapy appears as an effective form of therapy in psychiatric care. At the same time, it becomes clear that drama therapy as a research field requires further studies, which on the one hand provide deeper insights into drama therapeutic mechanisms and on the other hand, prove effects of drama therapy based on evidence.

Although the occurrence of drama therapy is growing in psychiatric care, it is, at least in Germany, not widely recognized. In addition, there is usually a tariff grouping of drama therapists, which is much lower than that of psychotherapists or behavioral therapists.

Studies in drama therapy help to clarify the principles of drama therapeutic practice, therefore they often use a qualitative design with case studies as an outcome. There is a growing number of qualitative studies in drama therapy, but only few quantitative studies, of which even fewer meet the standards of evidence-based medicine (EBM), which is the gold standard for evaluating and proving the value of a therapy. For drama therapy as a research field this means that despite the increasing number of studies the effectiveness of drama therapy remains to be proven.

Due to a prevalence of small sample sizes or the problem to find a working and meaningful control group, quantitative studies in drama therapy often fail to fulfill the criteria of EBM. Naturally in drama therapy studies a control group cannot be created in the same way as in medical studies where, for instance, a new drug is tested and the control group receives a placebo. What could a placebo for drama therapy be? The difficulty of transferring an EBM research design to drama therapy

S. Klees (✉)
Faculty of Environment, Design, Therapy, Nürtingen Geislingen University, Nürtingen, Germany
e-mail: kontakt@simoneklees.de

U. Volpe (ed.), *Arts Therapies in Psychiatric Rehabilitation*,
https://doi.org/10.1007/978-3-030-76208-7_23

stems from different basic principles underlying medicine and drama therapy, even if an awareness of a biopsychosocial model in medicine is gaining ground. While medical therapy aims to reduce symptoms, the success of which can be measured, drama therapy widely follows a psychodynamic concept of healing in which *new insights* or *psychological flexibility* represent basic therapeutic goals [1]. The question is, how can new insights or greater flexibility be measured as therapy outcome? Currently there is no satisfying answer to this question which points to the need for the development of adequate concepts to assess drama therapy outcome. One of the challenges that efficacy research faces in drama therapy is its complexity. Researchers who investigate "complex interventions" indicate that they can only be examined in a multistep procedure [2, 3]. The first step is basic research, theory building and clarification of terms.

As Sajnani shows, drama therapy developed in an interdisciplinary manner, in a convergence of psychiatric or psychotherapeutic procedures with theatrical and physical forms of expression. Due to their diversity, different drama therapeutic models and methods have been formed in the past decades. As a young research field, drama therapy is faced with the challenge of proving its effectiveness and at the same time having to create the theoretical and conceptual foundations for it. The current qualitative research projects contribute to basic research in drama therapy and clarify the need to discuss terms and modes of action, while the few quantitative studies take up basic findings and make a valuable contribution, to prove their effectiveness.

Research is needed to enlighten the fundamentals of drama therapy not only to gain access to EBM but also to make the concepts of drama therapy transparent and promote the disciplinary discourse. In addition to steps in the direction of evidence-based research which shows the effectiveness of drama therapy, further insights into its specific therapeutic mechanisms are required.

Sajnani indicates that working within dramatic reality supports people in processing emotional experience. Participants experience themselves and their stories in a new way or from different perspectives in a dramatic reality. In order to demonstrate the specifics of drama therapeutic mechanisms, the research field needs methods to describe experiences and theories to explain them. A suitable research system is provided by grounded theory [4, 5] which not only explores new research objects but also aims to develop theory (an example of which is provided in Cassidy's investigation [6]).

Sajnani mentions the need for mixed method designs, in which qualitative and quantitative procedures are combined and the necessity of studies that reflect the perspective of participants in drama therapy.

The author is currently carrying out a pilot project as part of her dissertation in which six drama therapy clients in a clinical general psychiatric setting were interviewed about their experience in drama therapeutic play processes. The interviews have been added by a 4-week observation of the drama therapy group. The aim of this investigation is to reconstruct aesthetic experience in drama therapeutic play situations based on the narrative of the interviewed. This research relies on a conception of aesthetic experience that is based on a drama educational model [7] which describes the experience of an "in-between," the "experience of difference" between actor/actress and figure or the stage, and the audience as core principle of aesthetic experience. The pilot study provides first indications of how an empirical approach to the experience of participants in drama therapy can be achieved. Therefore, a special form of interview, the dialogical reconstruction [8], was developed. More results of the piloting are pending.

Sajnani highlights that the future prospects for drama therapy are promising as it helps to support health and well-being of participants in psychiatric care. The developments in the research field are also encouraging and will hopefully lead to a growing recognition of drama therapy as a powerful therapeutic practice.

References

1. Cassidy S, Gumley A, Turnbull S. A grounded theory study of the processes that underlie change in dramatherapy: practitioners and clients experienced change in therapy through the use of techniques that created distance from difficult material, allowed clients to play and try out different ways of being and that encouraged clients to be actively involved. Arts Psychother. 2017. https://doi.org/10.1016/j.aip.2017.05.007.
2. Craig P, Dieppe P, Mcintyre S, Michie S, Nazareth I, Petticrew M. Developing and evaluating complex interventions: the new Medical Research Council guidance. BMJ. 2008;337:a1655. https://doi.org/10.1136/bmj.a1655.
3. Campbell NC, Murray E, Darbyshire J, Emery J, Farmer A, Griffiths F, Guthrie B, Lester H, Wilson P, Kinmonth AL. Designing and evaluating complex interventions to improve health care. BMJ. 2007;334(7591):455–9.
4. Glaser B, Strauss A. Discovery of grounded theory: Strategies for qualitative research. 3rd ed. London, New York: Routledge; 2017.
5. Charmaz K. Constructing grounded theory: a practical guide through qualitative analysis. Book. 2. Los Angeles: Sage; 2014.
6. Cassidy S. An exploration of the processes that underlie change in dramatherapy: a grounded theory analysis. Glasgow: University of Glasgow; 2013.
7. Hentschel U. Theaterspielen als ästhetische Bildung. 3rd ed. Berlin: Schibri-Verlag; 2010.
8. Klees S. Narrationen des Dazwischen: Dialogische ReKonstruktion von Erleben in der Theatertherapie. In: Ankele M, Kaiser C, Ledebur S, editors. Aufführen–Aufzeichnen–Anordnen. Wiesbaden: Springer; 2019. p. 295–312.

24 Dramatherapy: A Culturally Responsive Practice

Ravindra Ranasinha

Dramatherapy is a recognized profession in over 30 countries, and as per the focal article, licensed dramatherapists tend to work in four main areas: brief acute inpatient care, long-term inpatient care, outpatient care, and staff development. This reality differs, in the Sri Lankan context, due to nonavailability of a governmental healthcare monitoring body, to issue practitioner license, recognizing the practice, and the dominant psychiatric culture resisting psychotherapy, as "incompetent" for psychiatric rehabilitation. Hence, the dramatherapist is compelled to determine alternatives, to advance the practice, in Sri Lanka.

The current non-recognized status has disabled the dramatherapist, in Sri Lanka, reaching inpatients, and conducting staff development training. Private sector organizations, within their mandate, have been the support network, making the practice available for outpatients, and also creating opportunities to implement education and training in dramatherapy, targeting mental health practitioners. Some professionals attached to hospitals, namely, physiotherapists, occupational therapists, and medical practitioners, attended these trainings, gaining a broader perspective regarding this emergent field and experiencing active techniques in psychiatric rehabilitation. This process has increased the attraction of mental healthcare workers, towards dramatherapy.

In 2018, Mental Health Division of the Ministry of Health, Sri Lanka, organized a training in dramatherapy for its staff [2]. The Ministry selected 60 participants for the training, inclusive of medical practitioners, nurses, psychiatric social workers, and community psychiatric nurses. Training modules were designed to bring a high practical output. The modules included therapeutic games, improvisation, therapeutic storytelling, use of symbols and metaphors, therapeutic clowning, autobiographical narration, use of objects, rhythmic movement, poetry and singing, voice in therapy, clinical role-playing, use of mask, therapeutic performance,

R. Ranasinha (✉)
Research Centre for Dramatherapy, Colombo, Sri Lanka

U. Volpe (ed.), *Arts Therapies in Psychiatric Rehabilitation*,
https://doi.org/10.1007/978-3-030-76208-7_24

mindfulness-based dramatherapy, and conducting a dramatherapy session. Each session had the typical three-phase structure. This training was followed by supervision sessions, for a period of 6 months, to evaluate the progress.

The qualitative outcomes show that the use of active methods enables the practitioners and clients to form a helpful therapeutic relationship. Active participation of the practitioner, in therapy sessions, has been noted as a motivating factor for the client. Data reveals that in talking therapy sessions, clients prefer not to verbalize their difficulties and maintain silence most of the time. In contrast, clients have been able to use diverse objects, art, mask, music, guided imagery, and storytelling, as over-distancing tools, encouraging projection and self-disclosure. The results show that role-play, improvisation, playback, and performance, as under-distancing techniques, have supported creative resolution of client's psychological difficulties. As per data, dramatherapy has been used to support clients with major depressive disorder, impulse control disorder, bipolar disorder, adjustment disorder, and borderline personality disorder.

Literature related to dramatherapy in Sri Lanka shows that networking with churches, temples, schools, and corporate sector has enabled reaching outpatients with post-traumatic stress disorder (PTSD), childhood anxiety disorders, obsessive compulsive disorder (OCD), and depression [1–4]. A study mentions that role-play and dramatic improvisation were used to assess the condition of a group of children, presenting symptoms of PTSD. They were victims of the 30-year-old civil war, in Sri Lanka. Dramatic projection, dramatic embodiment, play, role-play, and improvisation have been helpful towards their recovery [4]. Similarly, several other cases of psychiatric rehabilitation, too, have been elaborated in that study, depicting the mild, and subtle natures of dramatherapy, enabling patients to explore their "psychological worlds."

In a traditional society, as studies show, a culturally responsive dramatherapy practice is of significance for psychiatric rehabilitation [1, 4]. Integration of spiritual teachings, and utilization of a wide variety of signs, symbols, and concepts pertaining to the belief systems, support the therapy, enabling the client towards exploring repressed subjective material. Also, the use of archetypes, in this process, helps the client, to regulate thoughts, emotions, and behaviors.

A recent case of trauma underscores the use of dramatherapy, as a culturally responsive practice. The participants were children (n = 35), and adults (n = 20), affected due to the Easter Sunday suicide attack, in 2019. Both groups had separate sessions, respectively. As they were from a Catholic background, picking up spiritual themes, worked best for them. Hymns, prayers, parables, metaphors, symbols, and archetypes related to Catholic faith were integrated with role-play, improvisation, storytelling, and performance, to help relieve their anxiety associated with trauma.

It was evident that Catholic hymns, referring to Jesus Christ, and liturgical music contained the clients, enabling them to regain their lost strength, and dispelling their fears. Since the destruction was ascribed to Satan, passing of a prayer, in a circle, was a ritual of *exorcism*. Parables from the Bible were a resource that paved way for an inner search, to make life meaningful. Integrating this belief system into a dramatherapy framework enabled the clients to achieve fluidity, to overcome trauma, and to reconcile with oneself, and the reality.

Creating a dramatic reality helped the clients to interact with the "invisible" lost ones. It was an "imaginary realm" that engaged them in "make-believe" play. Hymns and prayers were tangible modes to enter into that imaginary space. It enabled processing their thoughts and memories, building a connectivity with the lost ones, with one's self, and with others in the group. The make-believe state generated a play space, causing a safe and comfortable atmosphere, for them to "ground" and emerge from their trauma. The group generated a sense of having a social network with the norms of reciprocity and trustworthiness. It was this sense of supportiveness from the group that finally went into changing their life.

In summary, several reasons determine the efficacy of dramatherapy for psychiatric rehabilitation: (a) use of *dramatic reality,* creativity, and play space; (b) devoid of clinical labelling, and upholding unconditional positive regard towards the client; (c) requirement of a minimum number of sessions for effective rehabilitation; (d) qualitative development of "self"; (e) client-centeredness; and (f) culture-oriented practice. Education, research, and training in dramatherapy, targeting staff development, has enabled mental health workers to utilize dramatherapy for those in inpatient care. The current non-recognized status of dramatherapy is still a matter of concern; however, the practice has advanced despite challenges. The support networks, staff development programs, and the patient base are strategic milestones, for the progression and recognition of dramatherapy, in Sri Lanka.

References

1. Ranasinha, R. Dramatherapy in Sri Lanka: reflections of a practitioner. Dramatherapy Education and Research in Sri Lanka, no. 1; 2019.
2. Ranasinha, R. Changing the attitude of sixty mental health workers towards dramatherapy. Dramatherapy Education and Research in Sri Lanka, no. 1; 2018.
3. Ranasinha R. How schools abuse and fail children: dramatherapy to heal emotionally traumatized school children in Sri Lanka. Dehiwala-Mount Lavinia: Hare Printers; 2014.
4. Ranasinha R. Dramatherapy in Sri Lanka. Dehiwala-Mount Lavinia: Hare Printers; 2013.

MIX
Papier aus verantwortungsvollen Quellen
Paper from responsible sources
FSC® C105338

If you have any concerns about our products,
you can contact us on
ProductSafety@springernature.com

In case Publisher is established outside the EU,
the EU authorized representative is:
Springer Nature Customer Service Center GmbH
Europaplatz 3, 69115 Heidelberg, Germany

Printed by Libri Plureos GmbH
in Hamburg, Germany